Spirituality and the Autism Spectrum

of related interest

The Complete Guide to Asperger's Syndrome
Tony Attwood
ISBN 978 1 84310 495 7

Asperger Syndrome – A Love Story
Sarah Hendrickx and Keith Newton
ISBN 978 1 84310 540 4

A Blessing and a Curse
Autism and Me
Caiseal Mór
ISBN 978 1 84310 573 2

From Isolation to Intimacy
Making Friends without Words
Phoebe Caldwell
With Jane Horwood
ISBN 978 1 84310 500 8

At Home in the Land of Oz
Autism, My Sister, and Me
Anne Clinard Barnhill
ISBN 978 1 84310 859 7

Friendships
The Aspie Way
Wendy Lawson
Foreword by Emma Wall
ISBN 978 1 84310 427 8

Finding a Different Kind of Normal
Misadventures with Asperger Syndrome
Jeanette Purkis
Foreword by Donna Williams
ISBN 978 1 84310 416 2

Spiritual Healing with Children with Special Needs
Bob Woodward
Foreword by Dr Hugh Gayer, The Sheiling School Medical Advisor
ISBN 978 1 84310 545 9

Spirituality and the Autism Spectrum

Of Falling Sparrows

Abe Isanon

Jessica Kingsley Publishers
London and Philadelphia

First published in the United Kingdom in 2001
by Jessica Kingsley Publishers
116 Pentonville Road
London N1 9JB, UK
and
400 Market Street, Suite 400
Philadelphia, PA 19106, USA

www.jkp.com

Copyright © Abe Isanon 2001
Printed digitally since 2008

Library of Congress Cataloging in Publication Data
A CIP catalog record for this book is available from the Library of Congress

British Library Cataloguing in Publication Data
A CIP catalogue record for this book is available from the British Library

ISBN 978 1 84310 026 3

This work is lovingly dedicated to my friend
Matt Townsend, my parents Andrew and Sinead,
and my sister Catherine

Contents

Preface

Writing this book has been a labour of love. Whilst I accept responsibility for all that lies between its covers, its inherent worth must be credited to all those people with special needs with whom I have worked over the past twelve years. I can only hope that I have done justice to their narratives and that of their families, carers and friends.

Working with people with special needs has enriched my life beyond measure. They have opened up my mind and heart to the beauty of the lost and the broken. They have taught me the value of 'listening and learning' as opposed to 'talking and teaching'. They have afforded me the opportunity to shelve my cultural baggage and personal bias. They have brought me laughter and left with me anecdotes to treasure for a lifetime. I have been both touched and humbled by their courage, patience, integrity and humility. I feel privileged to have been given insight into their unique perspective. This work is truly theirs.

Working on this project has also allowed me to fulfil a personal ambition, in that I have finally managed to meet Donna Williams. Her influence on this work and indeed on my personal and professional life has been and remains inestimable. The profundity, beauty and warmth of her books and music remain a constant source of inspiration. I can only hope that this work inspires others to read Donna's work.

I would like to express my appreciation to all those who have assisted and supported me in the production of this book. I am indebted to all those I have worked with on the autism spectrum over the past number of years – I feel privileged to have been given insight into their unique perspective; to my colleague and friend Jackie Breakspear who assisted me with the editing of this work and for providing invaluable insights into the emotional world of those who live with disability; to my colleague and friend Judy Townsend for assisting with the editing of Adam's narrative and for her insights into the personal and social reality of those who struggle with autism spectrum disorders; to my tutors Professor Elizabeth Stuart and Dr Anna King of King Alfred's College, Winchester, for sharing their wisdom and knowledge and giving me the confidence to complete the task; to Dr Hillary Cass, Consultant in Paediatric Disability, Great Ormond Street Hospital for her suggestions and advice on Chapters 2 and 3; to Joanne Douglas, Chartered Developmental and Educational Psychologist for the National Autistic Society for her advice on the clinical accuracy of Chapters 1 and 2; to Dr Judith Gould of the National Autistic Society, and Joanne Neill at the Allison NAS School, whose lecture notes were an invaluable resource in the compilation of the tables in the appendices; to Jessica Kingsley for both her professional and personal support; to all the editorial staff at JKP.

Finally, I would like to acknowledge a huge depth of gratitude to all of my family, and to my friends Finn Essex, Mark and Martha Doyle, Brid Newham and Jan Berry whose love and support have sustained me throughout the writing of this work.

Introduction

My choice of title has been determined by my experience in the field of autism spectrum disorders. There is no such thing as a pure form of autism. The range of the autism spectrum is both vast and complex. Furthermore, there are many people who have associated conditions. Whilst they may not be diagnosed as having autism, their conditions include a number of symptoms that are normally associated with autism. In choosing the title of the book it has been my intention to include the experiences of both those on the autism spectrum and those who are considered to have associated conditions.

Much of my research has been centred around the narratives of people on the autism spectrum. It must be borne in mind that there are relatively few written narratives available. The first autistic narrative (by Temple Grandin) was published in 1986 and although a number of significant works have been published in recent years, none has focused either exclusively or explicitly on the spirituality of people with autism. I have also sought to give a voice to the non-verbal narratives of those at the lower end of the spectrum. Those who are non-verbal provide us with the greatest challenge, in that they call us to be advocates on their behalf. A genuine and sensitive advocacy demands we enter into a unique relationship with these people. The radical nature of this relationship in turn provides us with a genuine spiritual context. Thus, the spirituality of autism-related difficulties is a spirituality that includes the reality of both the carer and the person with autism.

The spirituality of autism-related problems is a liberatory spirituality, grounded in human experience. Human experience is *ipso facto* spiritual experience. In this work I have sought to explore the experiences of the person with an autism spectrum condition from a broad perspective. In Part One, the subjective experiences of people with autism are grounded in the objective findings of the various related professions. In Part Two I examine their spirituality from the perspective of the individual's struggle to come to terms with his or her humanity. In Part Three I explore the spirituality of those who can neither reflect upon, nor express, their own life experiences.

In my investigation into the inherent nature and dynamic of the spirituality of autism-related conditions, I have drawn on both the verbal and non-verbal narratives of those on the autism spectrum. I have also considered the voices of the relevant carers and professionals in the field. Narrative methods have been employed throughout this book, as they are the most effective means of depicting the subjective experiences of the person with autism in ways that are faithful to the meaning, or lack of meaning, they give to their lives. Narratives, be they verbal or non-verbal, reflect the emotional dimension of human experience, a dimension that is sadly often absent from the objective accounts of those who work in the field. The consideration of the life experiences of people with autism spectrum conditions and the process by which such experiences are turned into text is an important methodological issue. The process is further complicated by the fact that many such people are unable to communicate fluently in speech. I have thus used a combination of methods, all of which are interrelated and complementary. Interpretation and analysis are essential components of a working method that seeks to give a voice to both carer and person with autism. The grounding of the spirituality of autism-related problems in human experience suggested an anthropological approach. This is the most appropriate means of giving cognizance to both the everyday reality of the person with autism and the objective findings of relevant professionals and carers. I believe this is also an appropriate approach as, in my view, the most effective way of interpreting and analyzing the ongoing transformation that occurs in the relationship between the person with autism and their carer.

My decision to explore the spirituality of autism-related problems was primarily based on my experiences in the field over the past number of years. In the light of my experiences, both as a teacher and a residential care worker, I was surprised to find that so little had been written explicitly on the spirituality of the condition. However, during the course of my research, I identified in the writings of Jean Vanier, the founder of L'Arche, a spirituality that had striking parallels. One of the most significant features of Jean Vanier's spirituality is its radical call for an approach that is both contemplative and active. The 'preferential option for the poor', which is at the very heart of the spirituality of L'Arche, demands we enter into a radical relationship with the broken. This must be a relationship of equality. In such a relationship we must recognize the spiritual wealth of the broken and allow them in turn to lead us to our own. The spirituality of autism-related conditions is thus focused on human experience. Spirituality is defined as the spirit with which we confront concrete reality and the 'preferential option for the poor' is perceived as the most valid means of transforming reality and of entering into genuine communion with self, other and Wholly Other. The spirituality of autismrelated conditions is, in essence, a liberatory spirituality, a spirituality that seeks to give meaning not only to the life of the person with autism but also to that of the carer.

In this book I have given consideration primarily to three narratives. Temple Grandin was born in Vermont and is now in her early fifties. She was diagnosed as being autistic (Kanner Syndrome) in 1950. With the encouragement of a very loving and supportive mother she managed to avoid being institutionalized. In 1970 she graduated from college with a BA in Psychology. In 1986 she completed her PhD in Animal Science, and has designed one third of all the livestock-handling facilities in the United States, and many in other countries. She is currently an assistant professor of Animal Science at Colorado State University. In addition to her work as an animal scientist, she frequently lectures on autism. She has published over 200 articles on her work, as well as a number of papers on autism. In 1986 her first book, *Emergence: Labelled Autistic*, was published. This publication was unprecedented because it was the first time a narrative had been written by a person with autism. Her second book, *Thinking in Pictures*, was published in 1996.

Donna Williams was born in Australia in 1963 and grew up in a working class area. She came from a dysfunctional family and was often subjected to neglect, and to verbal and physical abuse. Although her parents believed her to be autistic when she was a child, she did not discover this until early adulthood. Like Temple Grandin she graduated with a BA in Psychology and later with a Higher Diploma in Education. She moved to England prior to the publication of her first book *Nobody Nowhere*, in 1992. For a number of years she has worked in a consultative capacity with parents, carers and teachers of children with autism. Donna Williams' three autobiographical works, *Nobody Nowhere, Somebody Somewhere* and *Like Colour to the Blind*, published in 1992, 1994 and 1998 respectively, provide us with the most remarkable and definitive account of the inner struggles of the person with autism. In 1996 *Autism: An Inside-Out Approach* was published, followed by *Autism and Sensing* in 1998. Her books, translated into numerous languages, have had a considerable impact on both the understanding of, and approach to, autism from the perspective of the person with an autism spectrum condition. Donna Williams lives in the Malvern Hills where she continues to write, sculpt, paint and compose music.

The third individual is Adam, whose involvement with this book began during a period in which he was going through the difficult process of being diagnosed. His narrative was compiled from a short unpublished book of lyric poems, *Falling to Pictures/Drowning in Words*, selected extracts from his diary and conversation with him. The written works offer a private biographical sketch that extends over an eighteen-year period of Adam's life. I have included in the appendices the full script of the lyrics that were relevant to my investigations. Adam is now in his late thirties and works with children with special educational needs. He is currently working in a small residential school in England. This school caters for a wide variety of special educational needs ranging from severe to moderate learning disabilities. Adam has responsibility for the communication disorder unit in the school.

Adam's narrative is significant in that it contrasts with those of Temple Grandin and Donna Williams. Adam was not diagnosed as a child, but after an almost twenty-year struggle to come to terms with his emotional isolation and loneliness, he was diagnosed as having a number of emotional, cognitive and social impairments that are sometimes associated with high-functioning autism. Adam's impairments are far subtler than those of either Temple Grandin or Donna Williams.

Although grounded in the clinical observations of the various professions, the perspective offered in this work has been primarily taken from the narratives of these three individuals with autism spectrum disorders. The perspective has also been coloured by my experience of working with people with both high- and low-functioning autism over a number of years. Furthermore, in my choice of narratives, I have sought to offer as wide a perspective as possible. I have thus considered the narratives of both high- and low-functioning autistic people, whose perspectives range from having an objective and/or emotional understanding of their condition, to the non-verbal cries of the more severely affected. The lengthy consideration given to the nature of autism and autism-related problems in Chapters 1 and 2 of the book was necessitated by the fact that the unique perspective of the narratives could only be appreciated if grounded in a comprehensive understanding of both the nature and complexity of the condition. Thus, the spirituality of autism-related conditions, as manifested in the struggles of the person with autism to come to terms with his or her humanity, is unlikely to be appreciated without an understanding of the controversial diagnostic issues which have been, and continue to be, associated with the condition.

Autism continues to be the most complex and controversial developmental disorder. Diagnosis and intervention require a multidisciplinary approach, which can very often result in disagreement among professionals. In the scientific literature, D.V.M. Bishop (1989) demonstrates this point by describing the case some years ago of a young boy examined by a number of experts from the various professions. Although all were experts in the field of autism, each put forward a different diagnosis. In the past, in the absence of definitive causes and/or cures for the condition, disagreement as to what constitutes high- as opposed to low-functioning autism, and debate with regard to the extent of the autism spectrum, many individuals with the condition were misdiagnosed. The precise nature of autism remains controversial, although with the increasing interest in and awareness of the spectrum, and the growth of the literature of autistic narrative, the situation is undoubtedly changing for the better. Recent narratives by such writers as Liane Holliday Willey, Edgar Schneider, Jasmine O'Neill and Kenneth Hall, to name but a few, have substantially broadened our understanding.

The second part of the book focuses on spirituality from the perspective of the person with an autism spectrum disorder. In Chapter 3 I outline the hidden face of autism-related problems by considering Adam's specific emotional and cognitive impairments, and the 'compensatory flow' that accompanies these impairments. It is only in the light of the above considerations that we can come to an understanding of his obsession with religious experience and the inherent nature or dynamic of his spirituality. In Chapter 4 we consider Adam's approach to, and understanding of, spirituality. This approach came about as a reaction to his obsession with religion, a reaction that was only made possible by the diagnosis of his autism-related problems.

In Part Three of the book I have tried to outline both the contemplative and liberatory dimensions inherent in the spirituality of the narratives considered. In Chapter 5 I have considered some of the principle features of liberation spirituality. I have here sought to demonstrate, with reference to Christian writers on spirituality, particularly Jean Vanier, that the spirituality of autism-related conditions requires a commitment from the carer that is both active and contemplative. Central to this commitment is the belief that all reality is sacred and steeped in mystery; a mystery to be embraced, not solved. In Chapter 6 I have given consideration to the narratives of the most severely affected on the spectrum. I have done so to demonstrate that relationship and/or communion is at the very core of the spirituality of autism-related conditions. When we speak of the 'spirituality of autism-related conditions', we are in essence defining the radical and unique nature of that relationship or communion. Thus, the spirituality of autism-related conditions is a spirituality that seeks to include the reality both of the person with autism and of the carer.

CHAPTER I

Autism – Towards a Definition

The diagnosis of autism or any of its developmental cousins, including Asperger Syndrome and PDD (pervasive developmental disorder), can be a very daunting experience for those being diagnosed, as well as for parents, carers and professionals. The world of autism is enmeshed in controversy, evident in the disagreement among professionals with regard to what causes the condition and how it should be treated. Our understanding of autism has been hindered by the myths promulgated in the media, myths that are very often encapsulated in films such as *Rain Man*, which received an academy award for 'Best Picture' in 1988. In this film, Dustin Hoffman's portrayal of the behaviour of the central character, who was considered to have Asperger Syndrome, was indeed typical of some of the behaviour associated with high-functioning autism. Yet not all high-functioning autistics behave in this way or have the characteristics portrayed, and many (indeed most) do not possess the savant skills portrayed in the film.

Our understanding of autism has been further complicated by those who claim to have found a 'cure'. Over the years various intervention strategies, such as those manifested in the TEACCH, Lovaas and Higashi programmes, have been presented as 'cures' by the popular media. Likewise, in the hands of the media, the success of techniques such as 'facilitated communication' and 'auditory intervention training' have often been overstated. Although all the above treatments have contributed to modifying the behaviour and increasing the learning potential of people with autism, none offers a definitive 'cure'.

In the turmoil of controversy and debate, the views of enlightened professionals and parents and, more important, the views of those with the condition, have often gone unheeded. Solutions have been, and continue to be, imposed that are totally alien to the cognitive, emotional and sensory experiences of people with autism spectrum conditions. Stereotypes have emerged based on a few of the characteristics of autism, and for many years little attention was focused on the real inherent causes or on the complexity of the condition. General awareness of autism consisted of a perception of a one-dimensional condition with little appreciation of its overall range and complexity, and the failure to appreciate this resulted in misdiagnosis, misplacement and inappropriate use of limited resources. Many now regarded as being high-functioning escaped proper diagnosis and were condemned to dealing on their own with a condition of which they had little or no proper understanding. In recent years the situation has improved and this is in large part due to the publication of narratives written by high-functioning autistic individuals. This chapter – and indeed the entire book – attempts to capture the unique perspective of those narratives in order to reach a better understanding of autism and of its psychic and spiritual dimensions.

The Autism Spectrum

Usually the initial diagnosis of autism is based on observations of the child's behaviour. Temple Grandin (1996) notes that:

> Unfortunately, diagnosing autism is not like diagnosing measles or a specific chromosomal defect such as Down Syndrome. Even though autism is a neurological disorder, it is still diagnosed by observing a child's behavior. (p.45)

It was as a result of observing the behaviour of children and adolescents that the notion of an autism spectrum emerged. The spectrum was understood to consist of a group of developmental disorders all of which are permanent and all of which share a triad of impairments. The triad of impairments is manifest in social interaction, communication, imagination and a narrow and repetitive pattern of behaviour (see Appendix 1).

The physician Leo Kanner was the first to identify and name, in 1943, a pattern of behaviour observed in young children as 'early childhood autism'. In 1944 Hans Asperger identified similar patterns of behaviour in older children and adolescents. Like Kanner he used the term 'autistic' to describe the behaviour he had observed. Whilst both Kanner's and Asperger's criteria form the basis of what has become known as the autism spectrum, it must be borne in mind that, in the light of modern research, the spectrum is understood to be wider than the syndromes originally described by Kanner and Asperger. New diagnostic categories have emerged in recent years and some now consider the continuum to extend from disintegrative disorder to PDD (pervasive developmental disorder). There is much debate and controversy among professionals as to what constitutes each category and also which categories should be included on the autism continuum.

Some professionals consider each category to be a separate entity, while others suggest that there are many categories that lie on a wide autistic continuum without a clear distinction between them. I have found the following categories suggested by Temple Grandin very useful in defining the possible range or extent of the autism spectrum:

- disintegrative disorder
- Kanner Syndrome
- Asperger Syndrome
- PDD – pervasive developmental disorder (see Appendix 1).

It has also been established that a number of other developmental, neurological, physical and psychiatric disorders share some of the symptoms of autism. Whilst the table offered in Appendix 1c is not exhaustive it does give an indication of some of the conditions that are commonly regarded as being associated conditions.

A Continuum of Continuums

Ever since the term 'autism' was first used by Leo Kanner in 1943 there has been a plethora of explanations offered as to what causes the condition, how it may be diagnosed, how we might intervene or even 'cure' the condition, and how we may discriminate between those who may be low- as opposed to those who appear to be high-functioning. Donna Williams (1994) reflects that:

> …autism had gone from being seen as caused by everything from possession by fairy spirits to bad parenting. From psychosis to emotional disturbance. From retardation to a

sleep disorder, and most recently as a developmental disorder occurring either before or shortly after birth that affects how the brain uses incoming information. There is a bit of truth in most theories, but the total truth is probably found in none. (p.8)

From my perspective and indeed the perspective of the parents, carers and children I have worked with over the years, the various theories offered have sometimes been nothing other than a source of confusion and frustration. Over the years I have observed the suffering of those who were misdiagnosed and subjected to treatments that were totally inappropriate. I have witnessed the arrogance of professionals, parents and guardians as they applied 'their solutions', 'their cures' and imposed 'their world view' on children whose cognitive, emotional and sensory experiences were totally alien to that world. I have seen the heartbreak and utter confusion of parents and guardians who were faced with the prospect of having their child institutionalized – parents and guardians faced with almost impossible decisions yet deprived of the proper tools of discernment.

The failure to appreciate the range of the autism spectrum results in nothing other than a failure to appreciate the difficulties of those who live with the condition. This failure is often rooted in a failure to recognize autism as an extremely complex developmental disorder and is very often manifested in the debate as to what constitutes the condition (and even more so where it is a case of clarifying what are the determinants of low- as opposed to high-functioning autism). In such a debate some will argue that autism is primarily an emotional disorder, others that it is a cognitive or information processing disorder, with the recognition that some form of sensory hypersensitivity and/or, occasionally, savant skills may accompany either. In my opinion autism is very often a complex mix of all the above and the primacy of one dimension over another (in the absence of a definitive cause or causes of the condition) is very often dependent on the self-awareness or subjective experience of the individual with the condition.

There is no such thing as a pure form of autism. Both personal and professional experience has brought me to the conclusion that autism comprises a continuum of continuums. Where someone is placed on the overall spectrum, or whether he or she is regarded as being low-functioning as opposed to high-functioning, is very dependent on where he or she may be placed on the underlying sensory, emotional and cognitive continuums.

Beyond Stereotypes and Symptoms

In attempting to understand autism I have sought to go beyond the symptoms that are commonly associated with autism. These symptoms and their numerous manifestations (as contained in many of the diagnostic baseline assessments (see Appendix 1)) are undoubtedly invaluable in the recognition of the 'appearances' of autism. They are, as it were, the first step into the world of autism. Yet we must go beyond the symptoms, beyond the following appearances, which are commonly associated with autism:

1. Absence or impairment of two-way social interaction.

2. Absence or impairment of comprehension and use of language and non-verbal communication.

3. Absence or impairment of true flexible imaginative activity, with the substitution of a narrow range of

repetitive, stereotyped pursuits. (Tantam 1998, p.4, see Appendix 1)

Failure to go beyond these symptoms may result in the conclusion that autism is some form of irrational disorder. To assume this is to fail to recognize the possibility that people with autism see reality from a different if not unique perspective. It is a failure to reach beyond the appearances to the reality of autism, a failure to ask why. In failing to ask the 'why' of autism we are in danger of losing sight of the inherent nature and dynamic of the emotional, behavioural, social, communicative and cognitive autistic perspective. In failing to ask why, we allow ourselves to be left with a fragmented perspective, a perspective where impressions become stereotypes, stereotypes become facts and appearances emerge as reality. The following are typical of some of the stereotypes that have emerged:

- 'Autistic people lack emotional empathy.'
- 'Autistic people lack cognitive empathy.'
- 'Autistic people lack a sense of pain.'
- 'Autistic people lack a sense of humour.'
- 'Autistic people lack imagination.'
- 'Autistic people are mentally retarded.'

If we are ever to come to an appreciation of autism and, more important, to an appreciation of the feelings of those who live with the condition, it is crucial that we go beyond the symptoms and their associated stereotypes. In so doing we can extend our knowledge beyond the labels and address the causes. For it is only in addressing the causes that we can progress from the 'appearances' to the 'reality' of autism and ultimately to move towards solutions; solutions that will not only enhance our understanding of the condition but also, more important, transform the lives of those who live with the reality of their condition.

Compounding Collections of Autism-Related Problems

In *Autism: An Inside-Out Approach*, Donna Williams points to the danger of seeing autism as a collection of symptoms and notes that if we do so we make the assumption that autism has but one type of underlying problem, when in reality, she says, it is a complex collection and mixture of a variety of problems.

> I don't see 'autism'. I see compounding collections of 'autism'-related problems. I see different adaptations to different types of 'autism'-related problems. I see different personalities dealing with different types of 'autism'-related problems. (Williams 1996, p.21)

Donna lists the following problems that she has both experienced and observed as some of the key underlying problems of autism:

Control Problems	Tolerance Problems	Connection Problems
compulsion	sensory hypersensitivity	attention problems
obsession	emotional hypersensitivity	perceptual problems
acute anxiety		systems integration problems
		left–right hemisphere-integration problems

From personal experience and the insight gained from researching numerous autism narratives, and even more important from my direct contact with the children I teach who are on the autism spectrum, I believe that the above analysis offers an invaluable key to the world of autism. It is not my intention to attempt to offer an insight into autism by considering the above associated problems in a chronological, clinical or over-systematic way. Nor do I intend to proceed from that which may be considered the most complex to the least complex problem. The severity of any of such problems is, in the first instance, subjective, and second, must be considered in the context of other associated problems that might accompany it as a result of compensatory effects. I therefore intend to present a broad perspective that will, I hope, offer some appreciation of the autistic person's struggles, regardless of where they may be placed on the spectrum. Furthermore, I hope that this will offer some light on the 'compensatory flow-on effects in people where a problem that affects one system of functioning will cause a weakening in another as it tries to compensate' (Williams 1996, pp.21-25).

Low-Functioning versus High-Functioning

Before we look at specific autism-related problems I would like to give some consideration to the nature of low- and high-functioning autism. Low-functioning autistic individuals are held to be those who present with the classic symptoms and are usually non-verbal or have very limited use of speech. Individuals are regarded as high-functioning, on the other hand, when they appear to be 'normal' – or perhaps more often 'almost normal', in that they often appear to be 'odd' or 'eccentric'. This view, whilst accurate (in a simplistic way) has led to the belief that low- and high-functioning autism are synonymous with low and high intelligence, with an acknowledgement that either may present with inexplicable savant skills, even though in reality this is extremely rare.

According to some practitioners, the term 'high-functioning' is, strictly, used to indicate that a child has an IQ over 70. Those children on the autism spectrum whose IQ exceeds 70 can, according to some theories, then be divided into those with Asperger Syndrome and those with a diagnosis of high-functioning autism (although this distinction remains contentious). Yet it must be borne in mind that some children with an IQ of over 70 fail to achieve their full potential. Sometimes their ability to function at a level commensurate with their IQ is impeded by their autistic difficulties. Thus, the intelligence of low-functioning individuals or high-functioning individuals, or indeed 'normal' individuals is not always reflected in their overall level of functioning. The perpetuation of the view that high- and low-functioning autism are always commensurate with high and low intelligence can lead to a position that denies those at the lower end of the spectrum the possibility of progress. Equally, it fails to account for the achievements and progress of those who, for a variety of reasons and circumstances, have progressed from low- to high-functioning.

The persistence of this view is very evident in the debates of those who argue for the existence of a 'pure' form of autism. Very often those considered high-functioning fail to fall within the remit of 'pure' autism and are dismissed when in fact their struggle with the condition may be in many ways as severe as that of the person with a lower-functioning form of autism. The apparent propensity of high-functioning individuals to function adequately in a 'normal' world must not be seen merely as a consequence of their ability to overcome certain aspects of their condition. Many high-functioning individuals have not in fact overcome the problems associated with their autism, but in certain cases their apparent ability to function 'normally' is   the result of a complex range of adaptations. Such adaptations very often come at the price of living, with extreme difficulty, according to the expectations of others. Reflecting on the struggles of high-functioning people with autism Adam writes:

> A life lost in the shadows of others avoids exposure but only at the expense of the loss of self-reflection. Without self-reflection there is no sense of a true self. The self is just a shadow dancing in the skin of numerous façades to the tunes of compulsion and obsession. Self-exposure may be avoided but this is hardly a resolution of, or reconciliation with, the complexity of their condition. (Adam's diary, 1998)

I conclude this chapter with a quote from Donna Williams. Her reflections on the issues I have raised in this chapter are the most perceptive and accurate I have yet encountered. Her observations are also particularly pertinent in that they challenge particular assumptions, assumptions that give rise to prejudice and injustice that often result in the convenience of exclusion or in the denial of essential resources.

> There are mild forms and more severe forms of the different types of autism-related problems but severity does not make one person have a 'purer' form of autism than another. ...some people appear to be only mildly affected by their problems because they have become masters at adaptation and managing compensations but, in fact, actually have a greater degree of impairment. They function at a higher level than their actual abilities to monitor, process, or

comprehend this functioning. Some people, on the other hand, appear severely affected by their autism but, in fact, have a very low motivation to develop functional adaptations that would help them manage what is actually only a mild degree of impairment. They function at a lower level than they are capable of monitoring, processing, comprehending or coping with. Some people ARE exactly as they appear and some people are not. There are people who identify with autism but have only one or two of its impairments and people who fall on the autistic side of 'normal' who have a range of autism-related impairments but have these in such a mild degree as to pass for 'normal' under most circumstances. (Williams 1996, pp.21–25)

CHAPTER 2

Autism-Related Problems

See the children of the bitter rain
Copybook pencil in a satchel of pain
Alone with tears as buckets of rain
In an ocean of drought
The children of the bitter rain

(Adam 1997)

In the previous chapter it was stressed that autism, unlike many other developmental conditions, is a very difficult and complex condition to define. I have already noted that it is essential to avoid stereotyping, to avoid accepting appearances as reality. When working with children or adults on the spectrum we are often presented with behaviours that may appear bizarre, and which can very easily be misinterpreted. Such misinterpretations have often led to accusations that people with autism spectrum disorders are very manipulative – such behaviour can appear to those who do not understand it to be intended to produce a particular reaction in other people.

In such circumstances interventions are often suggested which can, from the child's perspective, appear at best confusing, or at worst as a form of punishment. In the past I have witnessed children and adults with autism spectrum disorders, and who are both sensorily hypersensitive and hyper-emotional, being subjected to touch-like or other inappropriate therapies. I have witnessed children being punished or having privileges withdrawn because their actions or behaviour have been misinterpreted. A child with autism may appear to be actually enjoying bizarre-like or destructive behaviour and thus he or she is often accused of 'knowing what they are doing'.

Experience of working in the field over a number of years has taught me that the interpretation of autistic behaviour is similar to reading a clock anti-clockwise. We must be very cautious in our interpretation of the intention of an autistic person when they display a particular behaviour. From the child's perspective, bizarre-like behaviour is, in most circumstances, unintentional and is very often employed as a coping strategy.

Bizarre-like and/or ritualistic behaviour is but the public face of autism, an appearance, a mask to be removed. Consideration of autism-related problems allows us to draw the mask aside. In this chapter consideration is given to these problems at their most intense and pervasive level. The perspective offered has been drawn from personal experience but, more important, also from the narratives of people with autism spectrum disorders, particularly that of Donna Williams. Donna's narrative is of immense importance in that, as she describes in her books, she suffered from many of the problems considered below at quite an intense level.

Cognitive Impairments

Systems Integration Problems

Most people are multi-channelled in that the brain processes the input from the different senses simultaneously. Some people with autism spectrum disorders lack this ability and consequently are only able to process a certain amount of sensory input at a time. Children with severe systems integration problems can only process the content of one sensory input at a time. In *Autism – An Inside-Out Approach* Donna Williams gives the following description of the process:

> Jessica's brain works like a whole load of separate departments where the managers of each department do not co-operate well with each other, and they take days off here and there when enough of the others come to work. Jessica's brain works in 'mono' (working on only one track at a time) where so called 'normal' brains work on 'multiple tracks' (working on several tracks at the same time). (Williams 1996, p.43)

The consequences of this for the child is that his or her thought processes are not integrated. In severe cases the child may only be able to attend to one process at a time. The child may register what he or she sees, but only at the expense of disregarding what is heard, and vice versa. The child might be aware of his or her own body and body feelings yet, if asked to perform a simple task (such as touching an object) the awareness of his or her body must be abandoned if he or she is to function and perform that task. Similarly, a child may be aware of his or her own body movements, but be unable to keep track of and process another thought simultaneously. Ultimately, he or she may appear to be very forgetful or to have a very short-term memory.

These children are capable of being aware of and experiencing their own feelings but only at the expense of not processing their thoughts simultaneously. Thus they are unable to reflect on their own feelings or emotions when they occur. The child may be aware of 'self' or 'other' but seldom aware of 'self' in relation to 'other' or *vice versa*. Whilst these children may be taught to 'perform' socially, they have little appreciation of what being social really involves. Social interaction is therefore very difficult and other people are usually a source of frustration and confusion for them.

Communication can be extremely difficult for children with severe systems integration disorder. Just as they find it difficult both to feel and to think at the same time, they also experience difficulty with speaking and thinking simultaneously. Consequently, they may express or vocalize their thoughts only in their heads and, in severe cases, be unaware that the person listening cannot hear what they are saying mentally. If they do manage to speak their thoughts, they have difficulty responding to others, as while the voice is 'online' the hearing is not.

Communication is further complicated by the fact that children with severe and pervasive systems integration problems cannot process what they are saying as they speak. Donna Williams (1996) writes '...when Jessica speaks, she often can't process what she is saying as she speaks because her brain can't process what her own ears are hearing at the same time as she is involved in the mechanics of speaking' (p.44). The consequences of this for the child are that he or she may go way off track, repeat things over and over again, use inappropriate volume, pitch or pace, and speak in a combination of monotone or odd intonation. This ultimately gives the appearance that they have little interest in what they are saying and are unaware of the impression they are having upon the listener.

The inability to function consistently in an integrated way is also manifested in the behaviour of these children. Their difficulty with body awareness can result in their experimenting with parts of the body that they have failed to recognize as their own. They may as a result bite themselves, exhibit excessive hand and head shaking, or hold their breath. They like to touch things and experiment with textures as a means of determining the boundaries of their own bodies and identifying the source of their touch sensations. Their responses to being touched vary. They may either ignore or tolerate the touch of others or, conversely, reject it as incomprehensible and distracting.

Left–Right Hemisphere Integration Problems

Left–right hemisphere integration problems occur when the left side of the brain is not consistently aware of what the right side is doing and *vice versa,* with the consequence for children who suffer from this condition that they are not always immediately conscious of what they have seen, heard or done. Whilst they are capable of learning, it can take them a considerable amount of time to become consciously aware of what they have learned. This awareness normally occurs at a later date, when their thoughts or feelings have been triggered by something external.

I have had experience of working with a number of children with left–right hemisphere integration problems over the years. Jane was a child who, in my opinion, was typical of children who face this difficulty. She sometimes gave the impression of being unaware of, uninterested in, or confused by a particular activity that was taking place in the class. Yet, when the topic was revisited a week or so later, I was always amazed by what she had retained. One of the difficulties of requiring time to process information is that when that information is eventually processed, it is processed out of context. Thus the significance of the information is generally lost. Although Jane was able to store up a considerable amount of information (both central and peripheral) her inability to process it in its original context meant that she was unable to use it appropriately.

This was always very apparent when there was a change of topic. Jane would often use the information she had stored in a previous module as a means of answering questions on current topics. For example, having completed a module on Islam, the class moved to a module on Christianity. When asked who was crucified with Jesus, Jane answered 'Muhammad'. Similarly, she was particularly interested in foreign languages and knew the greetings of, and how to count in, five different languages. One was never sure in which language Jane would greet you, or in which language she would respond in Mathematics classes. This gave Jane the appearance of, at best, lacking common sense or, at worst, being intellectually retarded.

Jane also experienced considerable difficulty in accessing the information she had stored or experienced and, although she could give you certain facts, she found it very difficult to express how she felt. Although she was very prone to correcting others, particularly if they mispronounced a word, this was typically a triggered response rather than the result of conscious accessing. Jane's inability to connect feelings with thoughts generally meant that when asked to recall experiences she did so with little or no affect, or alternatively with a stored socially expected affect. She occasionally exhibited outbursts of emotion that were totally out of context. This is what she described as her 'silly giggles'. It was as though she were releasing an accumulation of unprocessed emotions.

One of the most striking features of Jane's left–right hemisphere integration problems was manifested in her inability to act, feel or speak as herself. This was evident in some of her echolalic and echopraxic tendencies – that is, her tendency to speak or to act as though she were another person. She had built up a reservoir of characters, some from real life, others from television and videos, which she used as a means of responding to the expectations of others. If, for example, she were annoyed with someone, she would address him or her in a very formal, stilted and cutting manner. This was affectionately known as Jane's 'Mrs Bouquet' voice.

Perceptual Problems

In diagnostic terms this is generally defined as 'not seeing the whole'. Perceptual problems are manifested in the child's inability to process the whole of what is seen, heard or touched. Visually, such children can only process segments of whatever they are looking at. They then form what amounts to a mental impression from this peripheral vision rather than forming coherent mental images. They thus define and/or identify people, places and objects from the fragments they initially observe. As a result slight modifications or changes can be confusing and a child may be confused about the identity of a person if he or she changes their clothes. Perceptual visual processing problems also render eye contact and body language meaningless.

Furthermore, children with autism spectrum conditions do not necessarily attach the same importance to different stimuli within a single modality. For example, when we talk to other people we focus our attention on the speaker and block out background noise from our consciousness, whereas the child with autism may pay more attention to either a background visual or aural stimulus that we would regard as irrelevant and/or distracting.

Aurally, children with such perceptual problems may only process fragments of what they hear. They cannot find consistent meaning in words or intonation and will generally avoid listening to people talking unless their sound patterns arouse their senses. In some cases they cannot consistently perceive their own voices. Thus they avoid using their own voices or simply experiment with various sound patterns. The inability consistently to find meaning in words can also result in children responding with stock phrases that they have gathered from listening to others speak. They will apply these phrases to a variety of situations regardless of the context, with little or no appreciation or understanding of the appropriate pitch, volume or tone that may be required.

Children with perceptual problems also find touch confusing. They find it difficult to process where they are being touched, or how they feel about being touched, or indeed who or what they are being touched by. They generally avoid the frustration of being touched socially and prefer touch that is pleasing to the senses. In the light of all these factors, they very often perceive other people as a series of fragments and this in turn impairs the child's ability to understand how others might feel or think.

The behaviour of children with perceptual problems often appears bizarre. Unable to find consistent meaning in their world they will often experiment with their senses. This can result in their flicking light switches on and off, turning taps on and off, experimenting with the volume controls of televisions or stereos, moving objects to and from themselves repetitively. In extreme cases they may bite, slap or choke themselves, or pull their own hair as a means of determining the source and limits of their sensations. They may also indulge in tapping themselves or the objects of their environment. Many like to touch both people and things and will investigate textures with their hands or rub their cheeks against things. I taught one child who liked to smell and then taste any new item of clothing I wore to class.

Children with perceptual problems generally require time to process information and this can make it difficult for them to recognize their basic needs. Often they will leave it until the last minute to go to the toilet or will fail to interpret hunger as a need to eat, tiredness as a need to sleep, discomfort such as heat or cold as a need to change clothes, or physical and mental abuse as a need to take flight from dangerous situations. In severe cases, even when needs are recognized, fulfilling these needs can also be confusing. Donna Williams (1996) gives the following example of the type of confusion children with severe perceptual problems may experience.

> When Jenny goes to the bathroom, she is confronted with three white porcelain receptacles: the toilet, the bathtub and the hand basin, all within close proximity of each other, all with running water and somewhere for it to run. Because Jenny often has difficulty quickly interpreting the meaning of what she perceives, she is sometimes as likely to go to the toilet in the bathtub as she is in the toilet, without realizing until later (if at all) that she went in the 'wrong' place. When she manages to go in the toilet, rather than the bathtub, there

is a white towel on a ring next to a white toilet roll on a ring and this poses the same kind of problem for her. (p.44)

Attention Problems

Children who suffer from pervasive and intense attention problems often present as being 'hyperactive'. The sights, smells, sounds, textures and sensations around them constantly distract their thoughts. They are robot-like in their efforts to comply with the distractions of their environment. They constantly move from one situation to another, obeying the various sensations that have caught their attention; consequently any form of sustained concentration is extremely difficult for them.

These children find eye contact difficult to maintain, and this affects their ability to think of the person addressing them as a person. Similarly, any expression of affection appears to have little effect on them, due to their inability to attend to the other person's presence. They are also very difficult to engage in conversation as their minds constantly race towards the distractions around them. Because of the resulting confusion they can interpret all forms of sound as language and are likely to answer a question or make a statement by mimicking the sounds of objects or animals, whilst remaining unaware that others will not perceive these sounds as language. This inability to hold on to a thought or feeling denies them the possibility of reflecting on their own thoughts or feelings, let alone those of others, and they can appear to be unaware of the thoughts or feelings of others.

For those children who have a degree of self-awareness, the inability to attend to their own thoughts and feelings is a source of frustration that can result in self-injurious behaviour. In an effort to close out distractions they may rock, jump up and down or run in circles. Dominated by feelings of lacking control over their thoughts, they may be sensitive to others trying to exercise control over them and are likely to engage in throwing tantrums. Their inability to concentrate may also affect their sleep, toileting and eating patterns. It is not uncommon for these children to sleep for very short periods or to rock in bed, which keeps them active enough to avoid the need to be constantly getting up during the night.

Thinking in Pictures

A number of children with autism appear to be particularly gifted in a specific area. These savant-like skills (such as the extraordinary ability to perform music, memorize facts, paint, draw, calculate, produce precise architectural drawings, reproduce everyday objects in very precise details and so forth) may often result from their overall ability to think in pictures. Temple Grandin (1996) summarizes this process when she writes:

> I think in pictures. Words are like a second language to me. I translate both spoken and written words into full-colour movies, complete with sound, which run like a VCR tape in my head. When somebody speaks to me, his words are instantly translated into pictures. …one of the most profound mysteries of autism has been the remarkable ability of most autistic people to excel at visual spatial skills while performing so poorly at verbal skills. (pp.19–20)

Temple Grandin's ability to think in pictures in such a precise manner has enabled her to use her visual spatial skills to become one of the world's leading authorities in animal science.

It must be remembered that not all people with autism spectrum disorders possess the same visual thinking ability as Temple Grandin. Furthermore, it must also be borne in mind that not all highly visual thinkers have autism.

> People throughout the world are on a continuum of visualization skills ranging from next to none, to seeing vague generalized pictures, to seeing semi-specific pictures, to seeing, as in my case, in very specific pictures. (Grandin 1996, p.28)

Emotional Impairments

Emotional Sensitivity

Emotional hypersensitivity is extremely difficult to understand, let alone empathize with. Most of us take the awareness of both our bodies and emotions for granted. Yet emotional sensitivity, be it hyper, severe or moderate can have a devastating effect on an individual and in my experience is the area least understood and attended to by parents, carers and professionals. Emotional hypersensitivity is particularly terrifying for the autistic child, as it removes his or her sense of control. Furthermore, the child can never predict when such occurrences are likely to take place as they are, quite simply, impossible to predict. For the child it can feel like being attacked by a monster from the darkness, as he or she is totally unaware of the precise identity of the emotion or emotions that brought on such terror. Even if names are given to such emotions it still remains very difficult for him or her to distinguish between different emotions since all are experienced out of context as a series of overwhelming sensations.

Emotional sensitivity has an enormous effect on the social life of a child. People can be perceived as those whose expectations and demands are ultimately the cause of the terror they experience. The emotionally hypersensitive child can develop not only an aversion to any form of affection, but also a fear of the emotions themselves. Such a child will also live in fear of being given direct instruction or being complimented. Compliments for a task can result in the destruction of the finished product, as this will be perceived by the child as a source of confusion and terror. To avoid having feelings, the child will avoid touch and any form of social interaction that might involve the expectation of him or her having to feel. High-functioning children often compensate by creating characters or façades that will respond to the expectations or affections of others. As a result, their responses are often stilted, expressionless, detached and impersonal.

The communication skills of emotionally hypersensitive children are also significantly impaired. Maintaining eye contact and listening is difficult and often the child will walk away in the middle of conversations if the emotional impact becomes too difficult for him or her to cope with. Emotionally hypersensitive children generally avoid contact with others and rarely initiate conversation. They can often be prone to staring into space for hours on end or mentally repeating things over and over again to lose awareness of those around them. Emotionally hyper-sensitive children often become obsessed with objects, factual information, machines and systems, cartoons and so forth as such interests do not demand emotional interaction. They also find it difficult to express their needs and as a result they may develop unusual sleeping, toileting, and eating patterns. In the light of the above considerations it is understandable that they appear to have little empathy with the thoughts or feelings of others.

Acute Anxiety

The type of anxiety at issue here is not caused by external factors such as neglect or abuse. It is an intense and pervasive anxiety state that permeates every aspect of the sufferer's existence. Children who suffer from acute anxiety often have little or no sense of their own body, or anyone else's. They cannot consistently connect with their bodies or comprehend their body messages or emotions. Recently, while working with a disabled autistic child, I observed her overwhelming fear of having the wheel removed from her wheelchair to be repaired. It was obvious from the level of her distress that she found it difficult to comprehend where her body boundaries began and ended. It was as though she identified the chair as part of her body. Hands (even their own) can be a source of alienation and fear for these children as they have little comprehension of how they are connected to other parts of the body. This can result in a fear of being touched or comforted physically when upset. Eye contact is also a constant source of fear as children who suffer acute anxiety cannot interpret or comprehend the expectations of others.

People are thus conceived as a source of unpredictability and their presence brings about a sense of loss of control. Likewise, animals can very often be a source of frustration and fear. In such circumstances it is understandable that any form of social interaction or reciprocity is almost impossible.

Change of environment and/or routine also robs such children of their sense of control. This can be manifested in a fear of any object or place with which they are unfamiliar. Children who may use the toilet in their own environment may be terrified of using a toilet if it is in an unfamiliar environment such as school or a public place particularly if it looks different from the one they are used to. Fear of social interaction and change of environment can also result in eating disorders. They may also suffer from sleep disorders and a fear of sleep and the dark is not uncommon.

When anxiety states are intense and pervasive this makes it extremely difficult for that person to concentrate, pay attention or reflect on their own thoughts and feelings. This in turn makes effective communication very difficult for them to achieve. It appears as though they have little awareness of the thoughts or feelings of others. Often when such children attempt to express themselves their anxiety overcomes them to the extent that what is said may be meaningless and lack expression. Their anxiety also affects their intonation, which generally lacks any semblance of interest or emotion.

The calming strategies employed by children with acute anxiety often result in what appears to be bizarre behaviour. They frequently rock, or stare into space, which can appear to be a form of self-hypnosis. When over-anxious, they can strike out at the offending object or person, flap their hands, or indulge in self-injurious behaviour. Finally, the ability to cope or overcome such difficulties is very much dependent on their individual level of self-awareness.

Sensory Considerations

Sensory Hypersensitivities

The response of children on the autism spectrum to sensory stimuli may vary from mild and oversensitive to severe and hypersensitive. Over the years my observations in the class-room have amply demonstrated the nature and extent of these sensitivities.

Liam was very sensitive to touch and could not cope with being touched. He generally wore a black leather jacket, which he insisted on wearing in class, as it appeared to offer him a defence against being touched. He found any form of rough texture, such as wool or denim, very irritating and would not wear them, preferring to tear them up to throw them at the person demanding that he do so. He disliked having his hair washed, as he appeared to have a very sensitive scalp and complained that the experience was very painful. He would not take a shower, as he was hypersensitive to the water touching his body in that way. He would have a bath, but would only wash himself with a very soft textured sponge.

The fear of being touched limited Liam's opportunities to socialize, in that he would not use public transport for fear of being touched. Similarly, he was terrified of most social gatherings, as even simple acts of social interaction such as shaking hands were a threat to his sense of self-control. Liam's fear of being touched was also very evident when one observed him in public settings. He would walk almost crab-like in public, as he believed that walking sideways offered fewer opportunities of being touched. When crossing a road at traffic lights or other designated road crossings he would always stand a yard or two behind anyone else who might be crossing, for fear of being touched. This fear of being touched resulted in his adopting the role of doorman at school. When leaving a building or room, Liam would open the door and let everyone else exit as a guarantee against being touched. In the same way, he was always the last to enter a room.

Christine was hypersensitive not only to the sound of others but even to the sound of her own voice. Even though she was very strong-willed, she found communication with others extremely difficult, due to her hypersensitivity to the volume and pitch of other people's voices. When she did engage in conversation she always spoke in a very soft voice, which was almost inaudible. Social interaction was extremely difficult for Christine, as she could not predict or tolerate any sudden change of noise level. Group activities were only tolerated if she were permitted to wear specially adapted padded earphones. On some occasions she would make a monotonous humming sound as a means of blocking sounds she could not tolerate.

Christine would not attend any social gathering she could not comfortably predict. She had an extreme fear of high-pitched sounds such as alarm bells or the sound of a baby crying and these often resulted in her throwing what appeared to be an uncontrollable temper tantrum. Due to her aversion to loud sounds, she preferred her own company and would sit in the seclusion of her room listening to music on her personal stereo at an almost inaudible level. Her inability to tolerate sound, and the emotional and physical energy she expended in avoiding painful situations, did not afford her too many opportunities to reflect on her own thoughts or feelings. Consequently, she appeared to have little empathy with the thoughts or feelings of others.

Daniel, like Liam, was very sensitive to touch. This was particularly acute with regard to the textures of certain foods. He would only eat baby rice and mashed bananas. Occasionally he would eat sandwiches, provided they were made with soft white bread and filled with either tuna or egg mayonnaise. He also had an aversion to certain smells and would throw a tantrum at the table if he smelt one of these. He was particularly sensitive to the smell of curry or mustard. His sensitivity to smell was also apparent in the classroom. When teaching Daniel, the only body deodorant acceptable to him was baby powder, and when both my classroom assistant and I complied, he constantly told us we smelled nice, 'like my baby sister'. On a number of occasions I observed Daniel holding his breath when visitors came into the class and it appeared that this was his way of defending himself against those smells he could not tolerate. On a few occasions I observed him spit shortly after visitors left the room, as though he were trying to remove the taste of those smells from his mouth.

Some people with autism are also very sensitive to light. In *Nobody Nowhere* Donna Williams (1994) describes her hypersensitivity to light as follows:

> I discovered the air was full of spots. If you looked into nothingness, there were spots. People would walk by obstructing my magical view of nothingness. I'd get past them. They'd garble. My attention would be firmly set on my desire to lose myself in the spots, and I'd ignore the garble, looking straight through this obstruction with a calm expression soothed by being lost in spots. (p.3)

Eventually this led Donna to lose herself in the patterns on wallpaper, carpets, leaves, flowers or almost anything she chose. Her hypersensitivity to light made life extremely difficult for her, as she was constantly being distracted or lost in a world of her own. Her ability to engage in everyday tasks such as shopping was extremely limited due to the distractions brought about by the colourful displays in shops. Fluorescent lighting is particularly distracting and confusing for those who are hypersensitive to light. It must be borne in mind that an autistic person's sensitivity to light may be a result of information processing problems – in other words, it may be a perceptual as opposed to a purely visual problem.

Some of those who are oversensitive to light, or who suffer from Scotopic Sensitivity Syndrome[1], or have visual information processing problems may now benefit from the use of tinted Irlen lenses. These lenses can manipulate the light waves that reach the eye through the use of various tints or combinations of tints to compensate for what was missing or they can filter out what the person was 'getting too much of'. Use of such lenses can have an enormous impact on both the perceptual and visual problems experienced by some people with autism spectrum disorders.

> Instead of looking from tree to tree and shrub to shrub, I saw one whole picture at once, one whole garden. ...I finally could do more than struggle to imagine an unfragmented whole. If only on one channel – that of vision – I no longer had to imagine. I could experience. (Williams 1996, p.90)

Behavioural Considerations

Compulsion

A psychological compulsion may be defined as an irresistible urge to act in a certain way, especially against one's wishes. The range of compulsions experienced may vary from very severe to mild. In the case of the former, compulsions are pervasive and intense and dominate every aspect of thought and

---

1   Scoptic Sensitivity Syndrome is a condition that is often mistaken for dyslexia, to which it is similar in certain respects. It is a visual perception problem that extends beyond reading problems. Headaches, backache, stomach-ache, migraine, inability to sit still while ready, a tendency to read in dim light, reading in short bursts, trouble with negotiating the steps on stairs or an escalator and so forth are some of the symptoms associated with this condition.

emotional response. The consequence of this to the sufferer is that he or she is unable to control his or her behaviour. The inability to control such behaviour leaves the sufferer emotionally drained. The child may feel helpless and indeed alienated from his or her own body, and this feeling will be accompanied by a sense of hopelessness, in that the child is so frequently blamed for their actions or expressions, as though they were intentional. The inability of others to perceive the 'real person' behind the compulsive behaviour gives rise to a feeling of being unjustly treated. At the same time, the inability of the autistic child to control such alienating behaviour can result in feelings of guilt and self-hatred.

Social interactions may thus appear to be a very painful and pointless exercise. Such interaction may indeed be a trigger for more unintentional compulsive behaviour. The possibility of interacting with others is further complicated when every attempt at sharing one's thoughts, feelings or actions is thwarted when one tries to express oneself with intention. Self-esteem is further eroded by the fact that people may often regard the sufferer as insane or intellectually disabled.

Autistic children who are aware of their compulsions may expend considerable energy attempting to stop or modify their behaviour. Such behaviour is manifested in destroying things, tearing clothes or paper, spitting, striking out at other people, or giving unintended impressions to other people. The battle from within may include attempts to stop the constant repetition of sound patterns and jingles in the mind, or to the compulsion to click the muscles in the ears, or incessantly grind the teeth, all of which make it almost impossible to concentrate. Sometimes even attempts at self-expression are prohibited as compulsive thoughts dominate intentional thoughts and the contents of speech are consequently lost. This can also result in things being said that are irrelevant and out of context. Furthermore, the expression, intonation and pitch of speech may also be lost in the battle of intentional self-expression.

It is hardly surprising that any sense of self, let alone other, is lost and/or deflated in such a struggle. All attempts at reflection on objects may be lost in the compulsion to attend to the patterns found in objects. The inability consistently to reflect on either one's own thoughts or feelings, or the thoughts and feelings of others gives the impression that the autistic person is unaware of how other people think or feel, or indeed that others are capable of feeling or thinking at all.

The difficulties outlined above very often result in bizarre-type behaviour. Frustration may result in self-injurious behaviour. Rocking, jumping and tapping oneself are often employed as a means of establishing a rhythm which in turn has a calming effect. These sorts of behaviours are in reality an effort to establish some order to thought and exercise some control over it. Likewise, attempts to establish order or control over objects can result in a compulsion to tap or spin things. These children are also likely to adopt a variety of inappropriate body poses or gestures, or produce a variety of unintentional sounds or sound patterns. Rituals are also very important as a means of establishing control and these can impinge upon every aspect of daily life, including sleep patterns. Once established, any departure from such rituals can bring with it the fear that breaking such rituals often appears to entail.

All these compulsions are unintentional and the ability of the person to come to terms with or overcome such compulsions is, in the first instance, commensurate with that particular individual's self-awareness. One individual's compulsive disorder may be less severe than that of another yet he or she may not overcome this disorder as successfully as the more severe sufferer if he or she lacks self-awareness. Lacking in self-awareness, the sufferer can perceive compulsions as their intended wants or needs and consequently does not experience the same sense of 'being out of control'. Intervention in such cases, no matter how well intentioned, can have the effect of causing even further withdrawal.

Obsession

An obsession may be defined as a persistent idea or thought dominating a person's mind. An obsession becomes an issue of concern when its intensity is such that it dominates the individual's interests to the exclusion of all else. Obsessions, like compulsions, can offer a sense of security, a sense of control in what can otherwise be a very meaningless and confusing environment. It appears that nothing or no one can compete with obsession, because simply nothing else can offer the same consistent meaning or significance. Unlike the unpredictability of the behaviour and actions of other people, obsessions offer 'a consistent, predictable and clearly purposeful and seemingly intentional direction' (Williams 1996, p.29).

Communication will always be centred around the obsession and, regardless of the context, one can expect the same stock of replies in response to questions, remarks or suggestions. The conversation of those children who suffer from such obsessive behaviour is likely to be limited and inflexible. The thoughts of such children are very often impaired to the extent that they are not able to respond to anything unless what is heard reinforces or challenges the obsession. Thus, when asked to converse, or say something, the total lack of interest is generally apparent in the expressionless, mindless, and compliant or flippant tone of the response.

Because of the dominance of obsession in their lives, there is little likelihood of their attending to either the thoughts or feelings of others.

Autistic-like obsession can also result in bizarre-type behaviour. Often removal from the obsession can result in tantrums. Meals, toileting and sleep routines can also be affected and, if the child is totally obsessed with an object such as a toy, that object will generally have to accompany that child wherever he or she goes. In very severe cases of obsession disorders the individual affected may need to be prompted when to eat or go to the toilet. Such primary needs can be perceived as secondary by the child when he or she is engrossed in a particular obsession.

The ability of a person to overcome an obsession disorder is (similarly to compulsion disorders) dependent on their level of self-awareness. Where self-awareness is apparent the child's obsession may be creatively employed as a means of extending communication with that child and thus enhancing his or her overall social and communication skills. Experience of working with high-functioning children on the autism spectrum has taught me that modification of such behaviour requires time and patience. To attempt to eradicate such behaviour suddenly in high-functioning autistic children causes great distress to the child and will very often result in the adoption of another obsession. Even greater caution is required with low-functioning autistic children as the emotional distress that may result, even in slight modifications to obsessive behaviour, can be immense and may result in total failure.

The process of diagnosis has been described as similar to the setting of a graphic equalizer on a stereo (Hilary Cass, Great Ormond Street Hospital, personal correspondence).

When assessing the nature and depth of the autistic tendencies of the individual, it is essential that we investigate fully a series of the cognitive, emotional and sensory difficulties that may be experienced by them. Each individual will present with different 'settings' on their 'graphic equalizer' or assessment graph. The picture that emerges allows us to determine whether an individual is high- or low-functioning. It also allows us to determine whether their autistic tendencies are primarily cognitive, emotional or sensory or, indeed, to what extent they are a mixture of all three.

In this chapter I have sought to outline some of the principal cognitive, emotional and sensory barometers that are employed as a means of determining the precise nature of an individual's autism spectrum disorder. Unless we learn to identify and understand these autism-related problems effective communication with the individual will not be possible. All the examples given above are representative of the most extreme settings of the 'graphic equalizer' and are thus pervasive and intense. Very often such pervasive and intense settings are associated with Kanner Syndrome or 'classic autism'. In my experience of working with high-functioning individuals I have found that they are less likely to suffer from the cognitive, emotional and sensory autism-related problems we have looked at to the same extent or intensity as low-functioning individuals. Furthermore, their condition may not 'appear' as severe, due to their ability to compensate for deficiencies in certain areas, and they are thus more likely to present as being 'normal'.

For parents, carers and professionals, living and working with the reality of autistic-like behaviour can be extremely stressful and confusing. It is only when such behaviour is understood in the light of autism-related problems that we pass from the appearances to the reality of the condition. In so doing, we afford ourselves the opportunity of being 'in empathy with' as opposed to being 'sympathetic towards' the individual. Ultimately, we can only gain insight into the spirituality of autism, into the struggle of the autistic individual to come to terms with their humanity, if such insight is grounded in the experiences of the sufferer and referenced in the reality of autism-related problems. Whilst autism- related problems are not unique to the condition of autism, and are shared (as we have seen in the previous chapter) with a number of associated conditions, nonetheless, an appreciation of such problems provides us with a genuine spiritual context – a context in which we can increase our understanding of the condition and, in the absence of a medical 'cure', in which we can assist the person with the condition in some way, however limited, to come to terms with their humanity on their own terms.

Finally, when considering the triad of impairments and the associated behavioural traits (in the light of autism- related problems) it is essential that we do not lose sight of the personality or the uniqueness of the individual. People with autism are as unique as any other human being. Research and experience have taught me that one can never fully understand or come to terms with the mystery of the autistic personality. It is virtually impossible definitively to trace or find the source of all the various manifestations of the triad of impairments and their associated behavioural traits in autism-related problems. For example, the inability to process thought and emotions simultaneously could be attributed to one or other of the cognitive impairments. Equally, it could be attributed to either a sensory or an emotional impairment. In severe cases definitive judgements are extremely difficult to establish.

'Autism' is spoken of by some people as a jigsaw with a missing piece. I experienced my own autism' as one bucket with several different jigsaws in it, all jumbled together and all missing a few pieces each but with a few extra pieces that didn't belong to any of these jigsaws. The first dilemma for me was sorting out which pieces were missing and which ones weren't supposed to be in my bucket at all. (Williams 1996, p.1)

CHAPTER 3

Coming to Terms

In the previous two chapters I have outlined some of the limitations of the notion that there is a 'pure' form of autism and I have argued that autism should rather be considered as a collection of autism-related problems. The failure to consider autism in this way results in a failure to recognize the more subtle symptoms of the condition. These symptoms, generally associated with those who are considered high-functioning, can remain undetected due to the compensatory flow that very often accompanies high-functioning autism – people with high-functioning autism are notoriously good at 'pretending to be normal', to use Liane Holliday Willey's expression, as they work hard to mask their external symptoms.

In this chapter I want to look at Adam's narrative. Adam is typical of many high-functioning autistic people in that his autistic traits are subtler and less pronounced than those seen in Kanner Syndrome or classical autism. Adam's ability to compensate for his emotional, cognitive and social impairments by the use of façades, and the subtleties of his obsessive and compulsive behaviour, are typical of the invisibility of high-functioning autism. By 'façades' I mean the ability to hide behind a façade, made up by the person with

Asperger Syndrome or high-functioning autism, which enables them to appear to be 'normal'.

Temple Grandin points out that many Asperger individuals are never formally diagnosed, and they often hold jobs and live independently. They function well professionally and their autistic traits are considered little more than oddities, eccentricities, or special talents. Yet, personally and socially, they can live extremely isolated lives with no proper terms of reference to enable them to understand, let alone cope with, their inner turmoil.

High-functioning autistic people, or individuals with autism-related problems such as Adam, are difficult to recognize because, amongst other things, unlike those diagnosed with classical autism or Kanner Syndrome, they do not suffer severe sensory scrambling and tend not to suffer speech delay at an early age. And, as I have said, are also often adept at appearing 'normal', so that although they may have trouble coping with the world, this is often not apparent to the outside world. Autistic children are often initially diagnosed as a result of observations made of their obsessive, compulsive, or ritualistic behavioural traits. Adults are more difficult to diagnose, largely because, if they have not been diagnosed as children, it is likely that they have found ways of coping with the world, albeit often with considerable difficulty. Temple Grandin goes so far as to say that the only really accurate way to diagnose autism in an adult is through an interview that looks in detail at his or her early childhood and, in addition, through getting proper descriptions of his or her behaviour from parents or teachers.

Working with adolescent children on the autism spectrum has brought me to the same conclusion. Temple Grandin's suggests that high-functioning autism can become more apparent or acute in adolescence and my experience fully bears this out. Whilst high-functioning autistic children can adapt socially and cognitively in their earlier years, they struggle with the emotional dimension of their impairment in adolescence in particular. Quite a significant number of those who suffer from Asperger Syndrome are not diagnosed until early adolescence. Adam believes that his autistic traits really only emerged and became an issue for him during his adolescence. Adam's narrative is, in his own words, 'not easily caught'. He is certainly not autistic in the classic sense of the term and would not be considered to have either Kanner or Asperger Syndrome.

> I am not autistic, at least not in the 'classical' sense as defined by Kanner or Asperger. I am considered to have PDDNOS (pervasive developmental disorder not otherwise specified). I identify with certain autism-related problems and have experience of their compensatory flow. They pervade every nuance of my existence. (Adam 1998)

In *Nobody Nowhere*, Donna Williams reflects that finding a label for her condition was crucial. Even though she had graduated in psychology and had undergone psychiatric counselling she had not been given a label for her condition. In a phone call to her father she demanded he tell her why she had been sent to a special school as a child. He replied, 'they thought you were autistic'. She had at last been given a point of reference, a key to self-understanding. Now she could begin to explore the confines of her inner world. Labels are only a first step, but a crucial one if we are to discover the causes of a condition and thence solutions that make possible reconciliation with both self and others.

give me a nail
to hang my picture
give me a label
for its title
then take your hammer
to my clouds of glass

(Adam 1997)

This reaching out for a label, for a means towards self-understanding and self-expression is also evident in Adam's narrative. In his diary he writes:

> A label is a doubled edged sword and I have known both sides of its cutting edge. Labels lie when manifested in misdiagnosis and you are subject to the turmoil of inappropriate intervention strategies. You are denied the right to self-access and the possibility of self-acceptance. In failure you recoil. You take two steps backwards before the possibility of taking one step forward. Labels transform to the extent that they offer you a key to selfhood. (Adam 1998)

Cognitive Impairment

In a way similar to that described by Temple Grandin earlier, Adam thinks in pictures. Yet his cognitive functioning is somewhat different from Temple Grandin's description. Adam thinks in what he defines as a series of images. He does not see in the same acute three-dimensional way as described by Temple Grandin and he certainly does not have the capacity to control his thought processes to the same extent. In psychotherapeutic terms he lacks the ability to control his free association of ideas. It is as though he cannot find a pause or stop button to control what he describes as 'a barrage of images and self-talk'. When Adam is tired, distressed or excited he can become obsessed with or haunted by a particular image or a series of images which will replay over and over again in his imagination.

Furthermore, these images are very often accompanied by incessant and obsessive talking. Thus, when intellectually confused and/or emotionally upset, Adam withdraws and will talk obsessively to himself for hours. It is, in his own words, 'torture by words and images'. It seems as though the process is a means of attempting to comprehend or express his thoughts or feelings, or indeed those of others. Adam also believes that his inability to refrain from rocking in his sleep, despite numerous therapeutic interventions, is also somehow related to his cognitive and emotional impairments. All the above defence mechanisms can prove very exhausting as they generally disrupt his sleep pattern. In the past this has meant sleepless nights spent pacing from door to door and wall to wall. Temple Grandin suggests that Prozac is very effective as a relaxant and observes that it reduces obsessive-compulsive disorders and the racing thoughts people with autism are often afflicted by.

Adam's specific means of processing thought has had an enormous effect on both his acquisition and interpretation of knowledge. He continues to find any form of abstract theoretical thought extremely difficult to cope with. He recalled that when he was at school, and later at college, the only way he could cope with abstract or theoretical thought was by memorizing it as a series of pictures. As he was unable to find mental images for all he was asked to comprehend, he designed his notes in a very specific format. He would then memorize the content as format as opposed to the thought contained therein. This was a slow and tedious task. Each passage to be studied had to be read numerous times before being broken into sections and labelled. The parts of the text deemed relevant were then underlined and the keywords highlighted. Adam would then copy all that had been underlined and highlighted into a note pad. He would then memorize the written script and reproduce it almost verbatim in written tests. If one considers that Adam does not have a photographic memory, is of average intelligence and often had but a limited understanding of what had been memorized, one can only conclude that the task must have been torturous to say the least. Yet this was his only way of coping with abstract or theoretical thought.

These procedures also catered for Adam's difficulty with sequencing in that the sequential order was already given in the written text. Sequencing his own thought still requires considerable effort. In his diary he noted that on one occasion a college professor returned a research paper and although awarded a pass, remarked that whilst worthy of an honours mark, 'the middle section should have been the conclusion, the conclusion at the beginning, and the beginning somewhere in between'. Adam holds an honours degree but believes that but for the fact that a lot of history is factual and can be concretized, he never would have coped.

Cognitively Adam also experiences great difficulty with concentration. This becomes particularly acute if an experience or a topic are of little relevance to him. In school he was forever being chastised for daydreaming. He gave the following example as typical of his inability to concentrate. In spite of attending piano lessons for many years he never managed to learn to read music or play in a classical manner. If he hit upon a sound that caught his imagination he simply drifted into space and was often lost to that sound for hours on end.

Consequently he could compose with ease but could never master the skill of sight reading or playing other people's music. Furthermore, musical notation, like mathematical and scientific notation, were quite simply beyond his cognitive realm. Sound could be experienced as a 'series of tone colours' whereas theory was but a 'series of abstractions'.

Likewise, Adam has little or no understanding of the workings of science. His difficulty in coming to terms with an objective perspective of reality permeates the whole of his existence. Indeed he has never felt the need to understand reality from an objective perspective. It is quite simply not an issue for him. He certainly appreciates the wonders and value of science but it has never occurred to him to explore its inner mechanisms. He simply accepts the basic laws of physics, chemistry and biology. It is as though his cognitive impairment has resulted in his unconsciously placing a mental blanket not only over scientific theory but over all theory, be it political, economic, social, psychological or philosophical. Theory does not often feature in Adam's grasp of reality.

If we are fully to appreciate Adam's spiritual perspective it is crucial we keep in mind his specific cognitive impairments and the particular way in which he processes information. Adam's view or understanding of reality is difficult to comprehend. On the surface, Adam may appear to be an articulate, well read and intelligent man with a very objective knowledge of reality in general, yet nothing could be further from the truth. What gradually became apparent was the subtlety of his cognitive impairments. In some respects Adam has remained cognitively immature. When one works with autistic children it is not uncommon to observe them taste, touch or smell the objects or the people in their environment. Unlike 'normal' small children they find it difficult to proceed to the next stage in their development. Thus they are very often over-reliant on sense perception as the primary means of accessing and processing information. This lack of cognitive development is often manifested in the difficulties many autistic children experience with reading, speech, comprehension and so forth, which in turn affects their ability to communicate and socialize. At the same time they very often seem to have what appears to be an instinctive sense of the real nature of other people.

Although Adam's cognitive impairments are relatively mild, it is evident that he continues to depend upon what he describes as 'having an inner sense of things'. Adam only reads when necessity dictates, as his brain very often cannot process the intake of both eyes simultaneously. To compensate for these cognitive deficiencies he acts out the thoughts and opinions of others in the various façades he has adopted over the years. Very often it is through these well-rehearsed characters or façades, behind which Adam hides, that he finds a voice that enables him to function in a social context.

He also employs a second and more subtle or hidden strategy, in that he will replay that which confuses him over and over again in his mind. This very often takes the form of what Adam describes as a video interview in which he imagines himself being interviewed. In the confines of his mind Adam acts out the parts of both interviewer and interviewee. These self-conversations are sometimes his only means of resolving both his cognitive and emotional difficulties. It is for these reasons that Adam, like many on the spectrum, *appears* to lack cognitive empathy and can very often only cope with objective reality on his own terms. Having an 'inner sense of things' may result in one having an unusual or indeed a unique perspective, but trying to interpret that which is sensed or experienced is an entirely different matter. In Adam's case, interpretation requires solitude and such solitude is very often permeated by obsessive self-chatter and a sense of isolation.

Emotional Impairment

you are a child
conceived in a tear
of loneliness
you sit by the water
the swell of emotion to hear
lapping in your soul
you ask
what is it all for

(Adam 1997)

Whilst Adam's cognitive impairments are moderate in comparison with those who are diagnosed as having Asperger Syndrome and extremely mild in comparison with those who suffer from Kanner Syndrome, his emotional impairment is intense and pervasive. Like Donna Williams (1992), he believes that autism has a significant emotional dimension.

> I believe that autism is the case where some sort of mechanism which controls emotion does not function properly, leaving an otherwise relatively healthy body and a normal mind unable to express itself with the depth that it would otherwise be capable of. (pp.181–2)

Adam cannot always process emotion in the normal way. Emotions are sometimes processed out of context and occasionally this gives rise to emotional overload. Adam gives the following description of the process.

> The conscious mind is now submerged; its submission inevitable. Slowly I subside into the abyss of nothingness. In the abyss there is no thought, no incessant inner chatter, just overload. Overload has its calling card. It emerges like molten rock. You fight the swell as it rises and falls. Every tick of the clock seems like an eternity. You feel it rise in the pit of your stomach and extend to your chest and head. The temperature rises. You feel its intensity as an inner blush. You fight in vain as your muscles tense. You find no voice for your inner screams. In extreme moments your blood pounds the base of your skull. Your heart races in terror. You stand naked and exposed. You have no name for this nothingness. It is simply an awareness of a terrifying presence. Momentarily you feel a chill as though your very soul is at risk. (I say soul as any awareness of body, of pain or of thought are momentarily lost.) The only consciousness is that of terror. When the terror subsides you stand amidst the ashes of "you know not what". In the ashes you are left with no solutions only relief. Inside you feel as though you have cried though you know you have not shed a single tear. In the absence of explanation or comprehension you stand without resolution. (Adam 1998)

It is extremely difficult to empathize with such emotional terror or fully appreciate the consequences it may have on the life of the sufferer. In *Somebody Somewhere* Donna Williams (1994) describes this emotional overload as the Big Black Nothingness and gives the following explanation for why it happens:

This was my emotional dirty laundry that had been stored up to the point of overflow. Too busy just keeping up with things, like a computer working to full capacity, there had been no time for emotions to register at the time I heard or saw or was touched by things. The feelings just piled up in the laundry room to be ironed out later. But life was too convenient without emotions and I kept leaving them in the room and the door would eventually burst open when the room overflowed...The tidal waves were my own delayed, out-of-context reactions. These terrible wailing bouts of Big Black Nothingness were emotional overload triggered by anything from happy to angry and everything in between. (pp.89–91)

It is with the emotional dimensions of autism-related problems that Adam identifies most strongly. It was only in the light of the emotional impact of the awareness of his condition that he began to realize that he did not process thought or cope with emotions in the same way as those around him. Although Adam is aware of an emotional inner-self that longs to reach out and be touched he remains unable to cope with any form of intimacy. He has never had an intimate relationship. When touched in an intimate manner it is as though 'my whole physical and emotional self disintegrates'. Adam is capable of both relating to and reaching out to comfort others but initially this was mastered by the creation of his façades. Adam remarked that since adolescence 'I have always reached out to others as "other", or a construed self behind "other", but seldom as self. To relate as self always involved risk, pain and overload' (Adam 1998).

This inability to relate to others can also be traced back to his childhood. Outside his immediate family, Adam has very little memory of relationships during his childhood. Most of his vivid memories of early childhood are of places or games he used to play. He simply cannot put a face or a name to a childhood friend up to the age of ten. Although he has had many friendships over the years most have ended in withdrawal and are now assigned to history. In *Preface* he writes:

> *Read these words as teardrops*
> *passing through the unknown depths*
> *to drown in pools of radical regret.*
> *Read these words as compunction,*
> *the compunction of one lost*
> *to the passing smiles of loved ones and of lovers.*
>
> (Adam 1997)

Adam's inability to cope with relationships also extends to his family and work colleagues. He finds it easier to keep in touch with family and friends by phone. At work he is thought highly of and respected as being a dedicated professional, yet he cannot cope with staff social gatherings. Adam's work is his social life. Although socially he lives the life of a hermit, no one either at work or indeed in his family seems to be aware of his total isolation. Adam's view of this is that although isolation is not a chosen option, solitude is preferable, if not inevitable, in view of his difficulty to relate to others outside of the façades that he has created. In his diary he writes:

> Welcome to my world. I have know it from the age of eight…My welcome is not extended without reservation. I reserve the right to solitude. I do not greet your attention. I do not greet your sympathy. I do not greet your touch, love, affections or expectations. I could not cope. (Adam 1998)

It is important to bear in mind that subtle or complex emotions can, as suggested by Temple Grandin (1996), very often be beyond the emotional horizon of some autistic people.

> My emotions are simpler than those of most people. I don't know what complex emotion in a human relationship is. I only understand simple emotions such as fear, anger, happiness, and sadness… But complex emotional relationships are beyond my comprehension. I don't understand how a person can love someone one minute and then want to kill them in a jealous rage the next. I don't understand being happy and sad at the same time… As far as I can figure out, complex emotion occurs when a person feels two opposite emotions at once. (pp.87–95)

The description of the range and depth of her emotions is typical of that which can be observed in Adam. Emotionally, there does not appear to be any middle ground or grey area for Adam. He is either totally committed or totally withdrawn, totally at peace or totally depressed. Mixed or complex emotions such as sentimentality just do not make sense to him. His self-imposed exile from social situations and personal relationships has often resulted in accusations of indifference. Yet in reality, largely out of respect for others, he strives to avoid social aloofness. His sense of isolation and loneliness is further increased when one considers the emphasis that is placed on relatedness and relationships in our modern popular culture. Furthermore, he continues to be perturbed by the petty deceptions he employs to avoid social and personal situations he cannot cope with.

It is important to keep in mind that withdrawal for Adam, and indeed for others who are emotionally impaired, is not a retreat into the bliss of solitude. Adam's loneliness is no different from that of any other human being. There is only so much of one's own company that any one of us can tolerate. Boredom is as much a facet of Adam's loneliness as that of anybody else's. Indeed, he himself defined loneliness on one occasion as a 'cancerous boredom'. Whereas most people may have the option of losing ourselves in the social company of others this is not an option for Adam.

Conclusion

Communication is very much centred around our use of language. The maturity of both our receptive and expressive language skills is very often commensurate with our ability to conceptualize. The conceptual process is in turn dependent on our cognitive ability to abstract, sequence, generalize and discriminate. These skills allow us to interpret language and make value judgements which will ultimately determine the way we think, act, feel or behave. Even non-verbal language as expressed in a simple embrace or hand shake is very often interpreted by way of conceptualization. This is our means of interpreting the subtleties of both personal and social interaction. People like Adam often do not have the same ability to process and consequently to interpret language (verbal and non-verbal). Adam's cognitive impairment, as manifested in the way in which he processes information, together with the attendant difficulties of sequencing, abstraction, generalizing and concentration, make conceptualization a difficult process for him.

Conceptualization is also an emotionally very difficult process for many autistic people. It must be remembered that people with autism do not have the same awareness of the subtlety of emotion as is the norm. I have already noted that subtle emotions and/or complex emotions are very often beyond their emotional horizon. Furthermore, I have also noted that autistic people may not appear to have the same range of emotions as is the norm. They are unlikely readily to identify with an emotion that is either foreign to their emotional world, or processed out of context. Thus, when an emotion is experienced, and later interpreted by way of conceptualization, this can be a source of confusion if that emotion is divorced from the lived experience.

Cognitively and emotionally the conceptualization process, be it receptive or expressive, can be a daunting and disorienting experience for people with autism or autism-related problems. Cognitive and emotional empathy are extremely complex processes. The ability of the autistic person to cope with such processes will be very much determined by, and indeed commensurate with, their position on the autistic spectrum. Low-functioning autistic people are less able to cope with cognitive, social and emotional empathy. It is simply not a priority for them in their struggle to process the most basic forms of information. High-functioning autistic people, such as those diagnosed with Asperger Syndrome or PDDNOS, also have difficulty with cognitive, emotional and social empathy. However, the latter group may be deceptive as they can be very articulate and informative, and indeed at times encyclopaedic with regard to issues that are of interest to them. However, one must not assume that empathy is beyond the horizons of all autistic people. Emotionally they can forge very close bonds with people, animals or issues that are of importance to them. Empathy is certainly possible for them, albeit at times very much on their own terms. 'My emotional empathy is limited; a one way train running to give, but never stopping to receive' (Adam 1998).

CHAPTER 4

Falling to Pictures/Drowning in Words

Earlier in this book I referred to the compensatory flow that very often accompanies certain cognitive and emotional autism-related problems. In the last chapter I described the nature of Adam's autism-related problems. I have tried to show how Adam's emotional impairments are pervasive and intense, whereas his cognitive impairments are relatively mild, with no evidence of the hypersensitivities that are normally associated with autism. I have also described some of the ways in which Adam compensates for his emotional and cognitive impairments. These factors have had an enormous effect on his spiritual perspective.

In trying to come to some understanding and appreciation of the spirituality of people with autism-related problems I have intentionally focused on Adam's narrative. Adam is in some respects obsessed by spirituality. This is very evident in conversation with him; when the issue of spirituality is raised his rate of speech increases considerably. Adam speaks about spirituality with passion. One can sense in the tone of his voice, and at times the unease of his body language, that his spirituality is a source of both comfort and distress.

This perspective of spirituality is of course coloured by the focus on Adam's narrative. All the same, it offers a point of entry into the spirituality of autism, particularly if we look at it in the light of Adam's specific cognitive, emotional and social impairments.

It seems that in the past Adam's obsession with religious experience was primarily an act of compensation. Religious experience provided a refuge from emotional turmoil, in that Adam interpreted emotions he could not process (or emotions he processed out of context) as religious emotions. Religion became an obsession and St Francis of Assisi the focus of that obsession. In truth, because of Adam's cognitive and emotional impairments, religious experience was reduced to a peculiar form of religiosity – Adam could not cope with collective experience or liturgy – and spirituality was understood as being synonymous with religious experience. It was only in the light of diagnosis, and the struggle to free himself of his religious and associated obsessive behavioural traits, that Adam would discover a far more fluid form of spirituality, a spirituality born of struggle and self-acceptance.

Collective Experience

they gave me words
they gave me walls
as empty as
alarm clock calls
my heart is flesh
my flesh is torn
my feet are tired
my bones are sore

you have denied
my child of soul

(Adam 1997)

Although Adam's spirituality was rooted in traditional Roman Catholicism the unique nature of his spirituality has been formulated in response to much of what he has experienced. Adam explained that, retrospectively, he had come to realize that he simply could not cope with spirituality when it was seen as the collective considerations of others. By this he meant that owing to the specific nature of his cognitive and emotional impairments he had found it very difficult to engage either in the theological and/or philosophical debate that occurred in the traditional construction of religious practice. Religious practice is underscored by dogma and cannon law and is consequently beyond the experiential range of one who struggles with abstract thought and complex emotions. Adam's cognitive inability to come to terms with universal principles and his emotional inability to share with others beyond the façades he had created, essentially placed him beyond the possibility of abstract religious and theological thought, and liturgical celebration. In spite of numerous attempts, Adam simply could not cope with collective experience. All attempts to come to terms with his spirituality through institutional religious routes have resulted in flight. Each successive flight was accompanied by an increasing sense of inadequacy and self-hatred. Eventually he would have to come to terms with and construct a spirituality that would accommodate his specific cognitive and emotional impairments.

Religion for Adam was a very personal affair and has in the past been a source of immense turmoil and pain. He speaks of religion in the same vein as he speaks about personal relationships. On one occasion he spoke of a 'lost soul violated and raped by the men and dictates of religion'. In view of his cognitive and emotional impairments, he has obviously experienced considerable torment in trying to reconcile himself with the inherent rationale of religion or religious practice, be it manifested in theological reflection or liturgical celebration. Moreover, it seems that in the past religion has very much been an exercise in compensation. It was as though he sought in religious experience that which he had so dramatically failed to achieve in personal and social relationships.

Adam now perceives involvement in both religion and theology, particularly in their ethical and moral dimensions, as a matter of choice. Such choice, is grounded in universal considerations that can be dependent on an ability to think in abstract terms. Religious belief and practice, in terms of choosing to act in a certain way, is very often grounded in theological principles. A grasp of such principles is beyond the scope of those who have difficulty coping with abstract thought or indeed of those who lack educational or socio-economic opportunities. Consequently religious faith or belief can seem imposed from above, imposed by an institution divorced from the reality and diversity of everyday reality.

The liberatory spirituality apparent in Adam's writing is in essence an attempt to reverse such a practice. Abstraction in whatever guise it may appear is, as we have already discovered, an extremely difficult process for low-functioning autistic people – but also for some who are higher functioning. Although high-functioning, Adam has an average IQ and is consequently far less able to cope with abstraction than those who possess a high IQ. Religious, theological and spiritual abstract thought is particularly difficult for Adam. In view of this it is apparent that Adam's choice to act or not act, at least in ethical and moral terms, have to be grounded in practice rather than theory.

Liberation spirituality places experience before the rationality of dogma and canon law. One is consequently informed by the deep experience of both individual and collective prayer as opposed to doctrine. Liberation spirituality is informed by prayer and thus maintains a crucial dynamic, in that it allows for the historical process to unfold in its admission that the spiritual experience of each generation, while rooted in the same tradition, may vary according to time and circumstance. Furthermore, liberation spirituality, with its insistence on the primacy of experience, also allows for the spiritual diversity encountered in a multicultural world. Thus central tenets of faith must be experienced before being rationalized.

In apparent contradiction to his inability to experience a spiritual life in the same terms as the majority of other people, Adam, in common with many other autistic people, clearly has what amounts to an innate sense of justice, and a strong inner certainty about his spiritual self. It is difficult if not impossible to account for this in objective terms, yet these inner certainties are very characteristic of people with autism spectrum conditions.

Adam no longer regards himself as a traditional Roman Catholic, at least not in the orthodox or conventional sense. Because of his difficulty in participating in, let alone making sense of, communal gatherings and liturgy, he does not practise in a particular faith. Yet his movement away from the traditional spirituality of the Roman Catholic Church came, as already mentioned, at an enormous personal price. Adam longed to be part of the Church. For over twenty years he sought to reconcile himself with the central doctrines and practices of the Catholic faith. Yet his conflict with the doctrines and practices of the Church was in reality nothing other than an expression of his inner conflict with himself, and in spite of the turmoil and pain, he always somehow knew that his struggle was primarily with himself.

> Mine is the struggle of a voice longing to make sense of itself and be heard among others. Mine is a voice longing to step beyond the façade of St Francis to be heard as self. Mine is the struggle of an obscure voice desperately struggling to free itself from the oppression of religious, musical and occupational obsession; free itself from the hidden melancholic comforts of obsession. A voice struggling to be free, if not loved at least understood, and if understood, if not by others at least by self. (Adam 1998)

In spite of Adam's emotional and cognitive immaturity he is a very compassionate man. His compassion is unique if not profound. It is the compassion of a mature adult who takes his responsibility as a professional, colleague, friend, brother and son seriously. Yet it is a very one-sided affair, in that, although Adam can give affection he cannot cope with receiving it. Here we are faced with the apparent contradiction of one who is mature yet immature.

Adam argues that this contradiction is really no different from that of any other human being. He believes that each human being is a contradiction in terms; all are engaged in the struggle to be human. This is what he perceives as the essence of the human adventure.

Temple Grandin (1996) also observes that 'people with autism are capable of forming very strong emotional bonds. Hans

Asperger…states that the commonly held assumption of poverty of emotion in autism is inaccurate' (p.92). In Adam's case it appears that his strong emotional bonds are tied up in occupational and familial commitments rather than intimate personal and social relationships. Likewise, his spirituality is rooted primarily, though not exclusively, in subjective as opposed to communal experience.

Theistic Considerations

Adam reflected that it had taken him over twenty years to realize that his religious education had led him to see the God of Christianity as culturally a God of words, a God of walls, a God of abstractions, a God constructed and restricted by the static rationality of dogmatic conservatism, a God imprisoned by the institutional and cultural bias. Cognitively, Adam could never conceive of a God in those terms. As I have already noted 'words and walls' had become for Adam a symbol of his struggle against religiosity, religious institutions, religious dogma, liturgy and religious abstraction. Adam passionately believes that if Christian spirituality, or indeed any other spirituality, is to be relevant for either autistic or intellectually disabled people it must respect the culture of those who live without the ability to think easily in terms of universality and abstraction. Life and death for Adam occur in the blink of an eye. To comprehend or wrap that instant in abstract notions such as creation, salvation, resurrection and eschatology is cognitively beyond him. Every attempt to do so in the past had resulted in mental and nervous exhaustion.

Adam's comprehension of transcendental reality owes little to theological or dogmatic speculation but is primarily experiential and subjective. Contemplation of the divine attributes is for him merely a waste of time – a form of mental purgation. Adam does not believe that God can be comprehended in human terms. God is simply the eternal source of life, the mystery of all mysteries. The God of life is the God of all world religions and, he believes, has in many respects been desecrated by them all. Like Temple Grandin (1996), Adam believes no one religion holds a monopoly of truth.

> It made no sense to me that my religion was better than theirs. To my mind, all methods and denominations of religious ceremony were equally valid, and I still hold this belief today. (p.190)

God is perceived by Adam as an eternal source of light whose rays penetrate all reality. It is these rays that give each living thing its mystery, the mystery of life. Because these eternal rays of light penetrate all reality, all reality is sacred. What is often considered to be broken, disabled or profane is in reality steeped in mystery. Failure to observe the hidden mystery in the broken, in failure, in the oppressed, in nature, is, Adam suggests, an obscenity. Such failure on our part is, according to him, a manifestation of our selfishness, greed, indifference and thirst for domination. God as a transcendent being, or more precisely in Adam's terms, God as an eternal force, cannot be captured by our imagination or imprisoned behind our 'words and walls'.

Although they share the sense of certainty of God's existence so typical of people with autism, Adam's view of God is less objective than that of Temple Grandin. Her view of God is grounded in logic and intellect as opposed to emotion. She could not accept God on faith alone. Like Einstein, whom she quotes, she believes, 'Science without religion is lame. Religion without science is blind'. Logically she regards a belief in reincarnation as more valid than a belief in death and resurrection. God is postulated as an infinite eternal force. He is that mysterious force which gives order and meaning to the chaos and randomness of reality. God in Temple Grandin's view is the ultimate source, foundation, or mystery, as is evident in the cosmological theories of quantum physics.

> It was quantum physics that finally helped me believe again, as it provided a plausible scientific basis for belief in a soul and the supernatural. The idea in Eastern religion of Karma and the interconnectedness of everything gets support from quantum physics... In nature, particles are entangled with each other. One could speculate that entanglement of these particles could cause a kind of consciousness for the universe. This is my current concept of God. (ibid, p.200)

Temple Grandin's concept of God is not static but dynamic. She believes that the mystery of God is forever unfolding and will eventually be unravelled by science. The thoughts and works that are left behind by each successive generation, she believes, achieve immortality, and if we destroy other people's culture we rob them of their immortality. She takes a very practical approach to her spirituality and sees her pioneering work in designing various types of humane holding chutes for cattle and horses as central to it. In her work with animals she is at one with herself, free of the emotional bonds and expectations of relationships. Through her work she experiences a sense of self-worth, a sense of her interconnectedness to the apparent randomness of the universe.

In a similar way, Adam sees his work with children with special needs as central to his spirituality. He says that, outside of meditation, it is only when at work that he is totally at ease with himself. When working with children, he does not have to cope with the emotional demands that very often accompany mature relationships. Adam speaks of being 'connected by heart to hearts that allow me to be the emotional and cognitive child I cannot step beyond'.

Christological Considerations

Adam's spirituality is necessarily grounded in the experiential, and it is crucial we appreciate the uniqueness of this spirituality in the light of his impairments. His autism-related problems have had an enormous effect on his relationship with others. Like many people on the autistic spectrum he does not experience 'other' in a conventional manner. When he reaches out to or relates to 'other' it is almost always on his own terms. Whilst aware of an inner self, he is unable to relate to others precisely as self.

In the past Adam had adopted John Lennon as the personality, the façade, the human voice or means of expression of Adam's defensive and aggressive inner self. He also found an image to express the warmer aspects of his personality. Whilst his spirituality is undoubtedly rooted in the teachings and life of Christ, he adopted St Francis of Assisi as the means of mirroring his spiritual personality. He regards St Francis of Assisi as the 'most autistic of saints', the saint who would walk naked in his defiance of convention and the expectations of others. The St Francis of numerous legends was undoubtedly rooted in his childhood imagination. Adam's St Francis was very much a man of warmth, a man who seemed always to be present and attending to the needs of others. Adam has little regard for the harsher ascetics of Franciscan spirituality or what he regards as the sometimes over-emotive aspects of Franciscan devotion. He simply acted as St Francis acted regardless of the consequences either to his health or personal circumstances. Both at home and in the world, St Francis could always be depended upon to elicit the right emotional response. Thus, for Adam, the teachings of Christ were very often acted out behind the spiritual façade of St Francis of Assisi. Both cognitively and emotionally this was the most effective means by which Adam could come to terms with both his own spirituality and that of others.

Adam's spiritual and social façades were as significant for him as Carol and Willie had been for Donna Williams, as she describes in *Nobody Nowhere*. Adam's struggle to come to terms with and indeed forsake the mirror image inherited from a Christian background is no less dramatic than that of Donna's struggle to abandon her mirror images inherited from Carol and Willie. Like Donna, Adam would have to shed the outer shell and replace it with an authentic self. What became very evident in our discussions was how Adam's struggle with his spirituality was in reality a struggle with the turmoil of his inner self. In Adam's words, 'the Jesus I had mirrored for twenty odd years was precisely that, a mirror, a fake, a sacred heart upon a wall'. For Adam, Jesus was not an objective reality but merely a projection of himself struggling to be free.

Adam always refers to Jesus as 'Jesus' and never as Christ. When this observation was brought to his attention, Adam said that he had always had and continues to have difficulty with the concept of a Christ. His Jesus is, and has always been, that which he associates with his childhood. It is an image of a man dressed in a splendidly simple white robe. 'This is the Jesus of simplicity, the Jesus of compassion, the Jesus of existential presence'. There is a nakedness and purity in his concept of

Jesus. Emotionally and spiritually Adam remains very much a child. His concept was not that of Jesus on the cross, nor of the Jesus of parables and miracles. When concepts such as suffering, salvation, communion and miracles were later introduced these brought with them responsibilities and commitments, and as such these were always on, or appeared to be always on, someone else's terms, Adam could not cope. 'With the expectation of angels and words I lost my presence in Jesus and Jesus' presence in me.' It sufficed Adam to experience Jesus in terms similar to that sought by Donna Williams in her relationships with other human beings. In *Nobody Nowhere* Donna writes, 'This stranger understood my language. He spoke it himself. He simply stayed within my company, being' (pp.150–152). She could only cope with others if their presence was unobtrusive. Likewise, Adam explains that his relationship with Jesus must in the first instance be on his own terms.

Adam told me that from his perspective some of the traditional symbols of the Church carried too much conceptual baggage. The crucifix was one such symbol. He struggled for years to comprehend the theological significance of the death of Jesus. Jesus' passion and death remains far less significant for him than that of people who have died of terminal cancer or starvation. Indeed, from Adam's perspective, Jesus suffered for three days which is, in his eyes, nothing compared with the suffering of the victims of the Holocaust or those who suffer from muscular dystrophy. Adam is clear that this is not a flippant or disrespectful remark. He has nothing but respect for those who accepted the mystery of Jesus' death and resurrection. He is at pains to point out that because of his inability to cope with abstract thought and universals, explanations offered by dogma were simply beyond him. The inability to comprehend and/or accept in faith the mystical extension of Jesus' death and resurrection as postulated in theological reflection remains a source of regret to him. Furthermore, Adam cannot relate to what he regards as the over-emotive devotional outpourings of certain schools of spirituality within the universal Church. The charismatic movement in his view is a liturgy for 'touch freaks'. He is equally intolerant of any form of fundamentalism and regards it as the expression of those 'vainly indulging in spiritual masturbation'.

A Spirituality of Touch

when his thoughts returned
he sang a silent psalm
of recollection
"today I have been touched
touched
as by the whispering of the trees
touched
as by the scent of dampened moss
touched
as in the cooling of the stream
touched by a stranger
who came to run her fingers
through my hair
anointing me in oils
with hands empty of intent
empty of conceptual abstraction
another lover
resting in the emptiness of wanting nothing"

(Adam 1997)

In conversation with Adam and in his writings there are numerous references to solitude and touch. Adam identifies very strongly with unobtrusive touch. The passages from the gospels that refer to unobtrusive or silent touch such as: the woman who touches Jesus' cloak (Mark 5:25–34), the anointing of Jesus' head with oil (Matt. 26:6–13), the washing of the apostles' feet (John 13:4–5) and the drying of Jesus' feet with hair (Luke 7:37–50) are very significant for him. Although he finds it very difficult to accept the loving touch of others, Adam has a strong appreciation of the value of reaching out to others. In his work he relies very much on touch. Sometimes it is the only way to relate to or mollify the distress of others, yet it must never be obtrusive. Such touch is free of 'conceptual intent, it is a simple touch of love or concern, a touch to indicate presence, and in so touching I am profoundly touched. I am connected'.

As we have seen, there is a parallel between Adam's use of touch and that of Temple Grandin. In both Adam's work with children, and Temple Grandin's work with animals touch is elevated to a contemplative level.

> I felt totally at one with the universe as I kept the animals completely still while the rabbi performed shehita... Time stood still, and I was totally, completely disconnected from reality. Maybe this was nirvana, the final state of being that Zen meditators seek. It was a feeling of total calmness and peace until I was snapped back to reality when the plant manager called me to his office. He had spent hours...watching me hold each animal gently in the restraining chute. (Grandin 1996, pp.204–5)

Adam says that when working with the more physically and intellectually disabled he too is very often lost in a world of his own. He believes that in reaching out to others by way of a simple comforting touch he also is transformed.

> 'The comfort that I seek to give is returned in silence. When mystery greets mystery as mystery there is profound connection. This is how I pass beyond the mystics' *cloud of unknowing.*'

Adam believes the *nirvana* of contemplation or meditation is very often at hand, and all approaches by way of 'spiritual ladders and ascending mounts' are, from his perspective, nothing other than a form of spiritual materialism.

A Spirituality of Solitude

as evening fell
he found refuge
in distant hills
far removed
from songs of failing lovers
from the incessant throbbing
of the crowds
he sat with the solitude
of the water and the wood
slowly falling
into silent meditation
he was lost
lost in the emptiness of wanting nothing

(Adam 1997)

Adam also identifies very much with solitude and silence. Jesus' agony in the garden of Gethsemane (Mark 14:32–42), his silence at his trial (Matt. 27:11–14), and his many retreats into the hills or mountains to pray (Mark 1:35) are of great importance to him.

Adam believes that it was during these times of retreat that Jesus contemplated not only the mystery of the Eternal Spirit but also that of humankind. The active life or ministry of Jesus must, he insisted, be understood in the light of his thirty years of silence. He interprets these years as Jesus' contemplative years. He believes that these years lived as a simple carpenter were also years of inner turmoil, the turmoil of a man reaching out to come to terms with the 'mystery of mysteries' and the 'mystery of self'. Without such a reaching out in silence and solitude there never could have been any inner reconciliation with either himself or his fate. Adam told me that it was the above passages that consoled him most in his own times of turmoil. He learned to accept his isolation and loneliness and saw it as part of the inevitability of self-transformation. Furthermore, it was 'a stopgap to my being bitter'.

Contemplation and Spirituality

Hear that subtle heartbeat
In the silence of your soul
See the mystic waters running
Feel the healing in their flow
Cancel words and reason
So inadequate and vain
And let compassion dance around
The ruins of a Saturday child

(Adam 1997)

Adam's spirituality like all spiritual narratives must be considered in the specific context of his emotional, cognitive, spiritual and social environments. Adam believes his spirituality is rooted, like that of all other human beings, in his personal, cultural and religious experiences. He comes from a very loving family and as such believes he initially inherited the contemplative dimension of his spirituality from his father and the active dimension from his mother. He perceives his struggle to be human since adolescence as no different from that of any other human being. Furthermore, until very recently he was totally unaware that his emotional, cognitive and social struggles were in any way peculiar. It is only with the benefit of hindsight that he now realizes how his impairments necessitated a specific spiritual reconstruction of reality. This spiritual reconstruction may have come at a price, but in Adam's words it is simply 'the rent of being human'.

Books were never Adam's forte; in fact he had only ever read a handful of books, some of which he had great difficulty understanding. Adam has never read the Bible. His knowledge of the Bible, particularly the New Testament, was acquired by listening to the Bible being read at mass and spoken about in school. Adam acknowledged that because of his inability to concentrate and to cope with abstractions, his approach to spiritual literature was very much a case of living something first and recognizing it later in a book. This was the only way he could cope with abstraction. Adam could only approach the abstract concepts of spiritual texts if he were equipped or armed in advance with 'existential images' taken from his personal experiences. Adam feels much more comfortable with books on spirituality now, as his life from his teens to the present day has been nothing other than a collection of such images.

Though Adam is unlikely ever to have an intimate personal relationship, socialize in the conventional sense or be comfortable with most forms of academic or abstract thought, he is philosophical about the past and the future. For him it is all a matter of 'compensation'. He has come to accept his autism-related problems, and maturity has given him the wisdom to celebrate them. He believes his isolation and loneliness have enabled him to empathize with the loneliness of others and as such his autistic traits are the cornerstone of his compassion for others. It was during these spiritual struggles that he also learned to meditate. Meditation by way of a simple mantra was sometimes Adam's only way of slowing down the barrage of images and the incessant talking to himself that are very much part of his life. The mantra was the key to the 'restive' dimension of his spirituality. Yet, much of what he had read in books on meditation in the past made no sense to him. Likewise the particular form of meditation recommended was often more aggravating than relaxing.

Adam perceived that the key to his spirituality lay in having an inner knowledge of himself. The key was unexpectedly provided in the pages of autistic narratives which in turn resulted in his seeking professional diagnosis. These autistic narratives and the subsequent diagnosis provided Adam with the 'key to selfhood'. It was, according to Adam, only in the light of these narratives and his diagnosis that he came to a comprehensive knowledge of himself as a person. This 'key to selfhood' allowed him to understand and consequently release the turmoil of the past. Adam had finally been presented with the first rational explanation of the turmoil of his inner life. He had at last come to identify his emotional and cognitive disorders as the source of his unrelenting inner conflict. In his own words 'the release was profound'. It was only because he had come to terms with this 'self as self' that he had been able to return to his spiritual books and meditation and make sense of what had touched him so profoundly in the past. Consequently, this new understanding of 'self as self' would allow him to construct a 'realistic spirituality of self'. Of his spiritual journey Adam writes:

> *Now, I am returning to myself a child,*
> *solitude's child,*
> *a child of solo resignation*
> *threading the thin pencil line*
> *of his existence.*
> *I realise,*
> *it was your silence*
> *I misunderstood.*

(Adam 1997)

Adam finds it difficult to discriminate between the terms 'spirituality' and 'contemplation': both are intrinsically linked. Contemplation for Adam is very much an encounter with mystery.

Contemplation of God as a pure essence, or of the divine attributes was, as already stated, a form of 'mental purgation'. Adam simply deleted him from the 'meditative equation'. Contemplation of Jesus on the other hand is described by Adam as an 'exercise of repose'. Contemplation of humankind, animals and nature is an exercise of perception. It is a means of sensing and appreciating their individual and unique mystery, their 'inner ray of eternal light'.

Spirituality is also described as an encounter with mystery. Yet this encounter is more practical in nature. Adam defines spirituality as a 'personal encounter with mystery' yet this encounter must be 'subtle and unobtrusive'. Adam explains that to encounter mystery be it spiritual, human or natural is in essence to embrace mystery. To embrace mystery must always be, in so far as this is possible, a selfless act. 'We must learn to greet the mystery without preconditions and be present to it without undue expectations no matter how broken or depraved it might first appear.' Central to Adam's spirituality is the act of contemplation that allows us to discern the beauty of those who are so often regarded by society as useless or ineffective. If we touch upon 'the mystery of the broken' we are in turn humbled and transformed. Adam perceives spirituality as an act of contemplation and, as such, it is both a restive and an active process. In the case of the former it is a resting in the unobtrusive presence of Jesus, a resting in the emptiness of wanting nothing; with regard to the latter, it is a matter of both recognizing and being present to the mystery of other in a selfless or unqualified act.

Conclusion

It is understandable how someone, in the light of his inability to socialize and relate to others as a genuine self, would seek alternative refuge in religious experience. Such experience would always provide a barrier against real intimate human contact. It has taken Adam many years to realize that 'a heart that could endlessly beat for others but not for self' would not find refuge in the 'shadows of religion'. Religious experience for Adam was merely a form of emotional compensation and would continue to keep him very much behind his emotional wall of glass, an outsider looking in. However, it was as a result of this struggle to express his humanity within the confines of religious experience that Adam constructed a spirituality to accommodate his specific autism-related problems.

Adam's spirituality is at the very core of his existence. He is acutely aware of both his own spirituality and that of others.

We have already noted that Adam's understanding of reality is primarily experiential or existential as opposed to theoretical or speculative. Spirituality, as a path to self-discovery, has been Adam's only means of making sense and indeed investing meaning in realities and relationships that were beyond his cognitive and emotional capabilities. Cognitively he has reconciled himself to the fact that dogma unrelated to his immediate experience will always be beyond his comprehension. Some of the central tenets of the Christian faith are thus inevitably bypassed. The Incarnation, the Resurrection, Salvation, Eschatology and the Trinity have played little or no part in Adam's comprehension of spirituality. Likewise, faith, hope, mercy, and to a lesser extent charity, carry too much conceptual baggage for him and consequently are reduced to 'the different movements of love'. Grace, from Adam's point of view, is both an awareness and appreciation of the inner mystery of self and others. It is not perceived by him as a gift but rather something that is earned through the struggle and turmoil of being human.

God can only be conceived by him as an untouchable eternal light whose rays give life and mystery to the whole of creation. He can only identify with the existential Jesus, the Jesus of personal and by extension universal peace. Contemplation of Jesus is achieved by way of a simple mantra. Adam has no expectations of Jesus, spiritual or otherwise; he simply rests in his company by way of non-discursive prayer. Meditative prayer is essential to Adam as it provides him with a means of stopping or slowing down the barrage of images and obsessive talking that he experiences as part of his emotional and cognitive impairment. Furthermore, it is very often as a result of the calm experienced in non-discursive prayer that he can rationalize and express thoughts and feelings that were previously confusing or of concern to him. He believes that if Jesus speaks it is always through the mystery of others or their work, or the mystery of the natural world.

One of the most distinctive aspects of Adam's spirituality is its conceptual poverty and/or purity. This is not to say that his spirituality is lacking in concepts but rather that the conceptualization process is, as with many autistic people, specific or unique to his way of thinking. It is as though he had unconsciously placed a mental blanket over that which, in the light of his cognitive and emotional impairments, he was unable to recognize or cope with. Confusion with cognition, emotion and hypersensitivity often results in the autistic person withdrawing into a world of their own. Adam, by way of meditation, has learned to transform these periods of isolation and this partly accounts for the contemplative dimension of his spirituality. Although his approach may be considered apophatic his spirituality is nonetheless primarily experiential. Overall it is a spirituality that effects a creative synthesis between the contemplative and active aspects of spiritual experience.

CHAPTER 5

Towards a Liberatory Spirituality of Autism-Related Problems

In this chapter it is my intention to look at a particular understanding of spirituality which I believe addresses the needs of both those who have autism-related conditions and their carers and shows how much each has to offer the other in a relationship of spiritual equality. This is an understanding that has been formulated over a thirty-five year period by Jean Vanier and those who live and work at L'Arche. It is a liberatory spirituality, a spirituality that attempts to give a voice to the aspirations of both people with autism and their carers. In the context of liberation, both are brought into a new and creative relationship. In such a relationship there is no dominant partner. It is a relationship of equality and mutuality, and its radical nature is clearly expressed in the Charter of L'Arche.

> L'Arche is an international federation of communities, based on the Beatitudes and founded by the Canadian Jean Vanier in 1964. Each community consists of homes in ordinary neighbourhoods where folks with disabilities and their assistants live together, sharing life in a spirit of mutuality. L'Arche believes that 'people with a mental handicap often

possess qualities of welcome, wonderment, spontaneity, and directness' and that 'they are a living reminder to the wider world of the essential values of the heart'. (Nouwen 1997, p.15)

The Spirituality of Liberation

The spirituality of liberation as manifest at L'Arche is primarily a Christian spirituality. It is a spirituality that grew out of, and developed alongside, traditional theology as a response to the deliberations of Vatican Council II (1962–1965) and the Latin American episcopate's reflections at Mendellin in 1968. Both Vatican Council II and Mendellin gave rise to a more comprehensive understanding of the terms 'spirituality' and 'liberation'. In view of the sufferings of the poor and marginalized, particularly those living in the third world, critical reflection on the everyday practice of Christianity emerged as a new and urgent task for the Christian world.

This was not intended to replace the two classic tasks of theology (theology as wisdom and theology as rational knowledge), but rather to forge a creative synthesis of all three. This synthesis is manifested in a change of emphasis, as is evident in the shift there has been from orthodoxy to orthopraxis. Orthopraxis is not a denial of orthodoxy. It is the means to balance and even to reject the primacy and almost exclusiveness which doctrine has enjoyed in the Christian life. Schillebeeckx summarizes well when he states:

> It is evident that thought is also necessary for action. But the Church has for centuries devoted its attention to formulating truths and meanwhile did nothing to better the world. In other words, the Church focused on orthodoxy and left

orthopraxis in the hands of non- members and nonbelievers. (Gutierrez 1996, p.8)

There are four things that have to be looked at in this attempt to make spirituality embrace the needs of the world. The first is the need to reappraise the meaning and practice of the spiritual life. The second requires an investigation into the role of reason in the light of Christian faith in a modern context. Third, there needs to be a critical reflection on the static ascetical-mystical spirituality or spiritual theology as traditionally practised, and fourth, arising out of the others, the development of a more accessible and inclusive spirituality. In brief, this shift of perspective is manifested in the transition from 'a static concept of spiritual theology to the more fluid spirituality' (Sheldrake 1995, p.41).

This change has brought about a deep questioning of some of the central tenets and practices of the Christian faith. Charity has been rediscovered as the centre of the spiritual life. Faith is expressed through charity, a commitment of oneself, to others and invariably to Wholly Other. 'This is the foundation of the praxis of Christians of their active presence in history' (Gutierrez 1996, p.6). Traditional themes such as eschatology, salvation, the historical process, human development and liberation are being re-examined. Equally, some of the central tenets of Christian dogma such as the Incarnation, the Trinity and so forth are being re-appraised.

This is taking place as a means of determining a more authentic form of Christian life, particularly when faced with the scandal of poverty and oppression suffered by the majority of the population in the third world. However, the move towards a radical form of liberation is not limited to third world countries. Liberation spirituality offers a voice to oppressed and marginalized peoples in every walk of life. Over the past thirty-five years a host of liberation spiritualities, such as feminist spirituality, gay spirituality and so forth have developed. It is in this context that the spirituality of L'Arche has emerged.

Living with Spirit

Throughout Christian history spirituality (that is, the theory and practice of the Christian life) has evolved and undergone many changes. The spirituality of liberation is traditional to the extent that it embraces and expands certain aspects of the notion of the spiritual life as manifested in Pauline and patristic theology. As in Pauline and patristic theology 'life in the Spirit' or 'living with Spirit' is a central and fundamental theme of the spirituality of liberation. It is precisely this life in the Spirit that enables us to, 'Answer for the truth of history truthfully. Shape that history, do not be dominated by it or merely slip and slide passively through it' (Sobrino 1993). This, 'being-human-with-spirit' allows us to respond creatively to concrete reality and transform that reality particularly with regard to the lives of the most marginalized and oppressed of society. Every human being is vested with spirit and has a spiritual life. Spirituality may therefore be defined as the spirit with which we confront reality.

> It is being-human-with-spirit, which responds to the elements of crisis and promise residing in concrete reality, unifying the various elements of a response to that reality in such a way that the latter may be definitively a reality more of promise than of crisis – that we call spirituality. (Sobrino 1993)

Although Christian praxis is a central theme of the spirituality of liberation, it is incapable of unifying the diverse elements of theory and practice, faith and reason, doctrine and administration. Life in the Spirit is the fundamental and synthetic principle of liberation spirituality. Jean Vanier (1996) writes:

> In order to walk with the poor we need to find strength, a new energy, not from books and studies or the need to prove something, not even from natural generosity and the need to grow, nor from the desire to save the world, but an energy which comes directly from God. We must be reborn in love and in the Spirit. (p.114)

An encounter with Spirit is neither abstract nor systematic. It is an encounter not only with a transcendent Absolute but also with an immanent God, present and active in human history. This encounter with Spirit is initially a subjective experience of spirit that very often occurs in times of crisis or uncertainty. The subjective experience of spirit is the means by which we recognize and respond to the challenging face of God as it emerges in the context of historical reality. Here, God is not postulated in terms of speculative Platonic or Aristotelian categories, but is rather seen as an event of meaning, of hope, of transformation and ultimately of liberation. All change, be it political, social or historical, has ultimate meaning only in so far as it proceeds from the mystery of God. In other words, the meaning and relevancy of God is best understood in the context whereby God is taken to be the 'only radically important piece of a given reality' (Boff 1992).

The God of Christian revelation is a God incarnate, a God present and active in all dimensions of reality. Contemporary spirituality acknowledges and expresses the incarnational aspect of faith, to the extent that we act selflessly on behalf of others, and respect the environment we share with others. All of reality must be seen, not in traditional terms of sacred or profane, but as sacramental. All of reality manifests the divine reality.

> Seen as a whole, the direction of theological thinking has been characterised by a transference away from attention to the being *per se* of supernatural realities, and toward attention to their relationship with man, with the world, and with the problems and affirmations of all those who for us represent the *Other*. (Gutierrez 1996, p.6)

This is not a static but rather a dynamic principle, in that every generation will have to face the challenge of recognizing and responding to God's new manifestation as it occurs in their particular historical reality. This spiritual collision with the face of God, particularly as manifested in the needs of the poor and marginalized is the basic challenge of the spirituality of liberation.

> The required activity holds a clear liberation dimension sprung from the incarnation of a Christian faith that now seeks to cling to the Lord of the poor. To struggle at the side of the poor, to be enfleshed in their longings, to commune with Christ present in the poor is to live in Christ's discipleship. (Boff 1992, pp.236-243)

Preferential Option for the Poor

Whilst a contemplative attitude is inherent in, and essential to, the spirituality of liberation, it must, on the other hand, be realized existentially. It must take a concrete form in action. This is what is realized in the 'preferential option for the poor'.

These people represent what Philip Sheldrake (1995) defines as the 'underside of history'. Until recent decades, these oppressed and marginalized peoples have never had a voice in either society or the Church. The spirituality of liberation is insistent that the poor be the locus of contemplation. God's predilection for the poor throughout history has prioritized their presence and struggles as the sacrament of his self-communication. The mystery of God's hidden presence in history is located in the poor. The 'preferential option for the poor' is a call to this presence and a call to action. It is a simultaneous call to contemplation and liberation, the latter implying political, social, historical and transforming action. This call gives us a view of the poor that is more than socioanalytic. Over and above identifying the mechanisms of their impoverishment, we are called to act with and on behalf of the poor. We must become enfleshed in their struggles and sufferings, open to their voice, their culture, their wisdom, and ultimately their holiness. In spite of their impoverishment, the poor have an innate and unique wealth of their own.

> People who are powerless and vulnerable attract what is most beautiful and most luminous in those who are stronger: They call them to be compassionate, to love intelligently, and not only in a sentimental way. Those who are weak help those who are more capable to discover their own humanity and to leave the world of competition in order to put their energies at the service of love, justice and peace. The weak teach the strong to accept and integrate the weakness and brokenness of their own lives which they often hide behind masks. (Vanier 1997, p.2)

Conclusion

The spirituality of liberation is primarily experiential in nature. 'When viewed in this broad sense of the term, spirituality is used to describe an element in human experience precisely as experience and precisely as human' (Downey 1997, p.14). Yet we must approach the spiritual dimension of human experience with caution. In the latter part of the twentieth century, investigations into the workings of the psyche, and our perceptions of the different levels of consciousness, have given rise to a plethora of psychoanalytic and psychotherapeutic procedures. In a rush to authenticate or validate experience we have, to a large extent, become what William McNamara (1991) describes as 'psychoidolaters'. Consequently, spiritual experience is often synonymous with self-experience, self-fixation, self-help. Spiritual experience is thereby impoverished in that it is reduced to, and expressed in, solipsistic and esoteric terms. If we are to approach spirituality holistically, and determine its inherent value, it is crucial that we identify the egocentric dimensions so prevalent and so detrimental to our culture today. If the self is to avoid the inauthentic solipsistic and esoteric expressions of the postmodern era, it must extend beyond the realms of self. Like the serpent, we must continually shed the skin of self if we are to enter the 'narrow door' and walk the spiritual path. This transformation of self is not a static process but an ongoing discourse or communion with others. This inter-subjective element of spirituality is crucial if we are to develop a selfless, as opposed to a selfish, form of spirituality. Authentic inter-subjective discourse and communion, as realized in the 'preferential option for the poor', are the indispensable dimensions of an existentially relevant and genuine spirituality.

In this chapter, I have sought to show how the spirituality of liberation carries with it a contemplative attitude. From my experience of working with those on the autism spectrum, I have found that this attitude is born out of a deep experiential relationship with them. Jesus' response to reality was as a result of this contemplative attitude. This enabled him to make the ultimate response to reality. Jesus acted with spirit and responded to reality with compassion. Although those on the autism spectrum, as the poor, may be considered as the locus of contemplation, they must not be used merely as a means of realizing union with God. 'Christ identifies with the poor in order to be served and welcomed precisely in them' (Boff 1992). Contemplation completes in liberating action. This act of contemplation instils in us the spirit with which we confront, transform and transcend concrete reality. The spiritual experience of contemplation and liberation thus restores the unity of faith and life, prayer and action, and spirituality and politics.

CHAPTER 6

Unqualified Existential Presence

How then to approach the miserable child
not haughtily
but humbly
not judging but loving
determined not to dominate
not even to give things
rather to give myself
my time
energy
and heart

(Vanier 1997a, p.4)

In Chapter 4 we looked at Adam's spiritual perspective. However, we have to remember that Adam's perspective, like those of Temple Grandin and Donna Williams, is representative of someone who is capable of both self-reflection and self-expression. For those whose autism-related problems are pervasive and severe, those who are considered to be at the lower end of the autism spectrum, such self-reflection and self-expression is very limited, if indeed possible at all. Yet, spirituality, particularly in its liberatory dimensions, is very much dependent on the voices of those who are so often ignored. The greatest challenge facing those who work with and care for people with autism is that of listening to, and giving voice to, the muted and very often non-verbal cries they encounter daily. Such a challenge demands a radical approach, an approach that places those considered the 'least' at the very core of our approach to, and understanding of, both our own spirituality and that of others.

In 1994 I took a break from the teaching profession and worked in a number of social care settings in London. It was while I was working as a residential care worker in London that my life was enriched in a way I would never have believed possible. In the short time I spent working with adults with severe autism-related conditions, I discovered the inherent and vital dynamic of spirituality. I was given a key to unlock the mystery of my struggle to come to terms with my own humanity and that of others. My life was transformed and profoundly enriched by the very people I had come to serve. In spite of their pain and the circumstances in which they were forced to live, these ten adults touched my life in a most fundamental and radical way. I can still remember not only their names, faces, likes, dislikes and personal histories, but strangely enough their physical touch.

All these young men and women were between the ages of twenty and thirty-five. The community, or 'clients' as they were invariably called, comprised four women and six men. Four of these people were white and six were from an Afro-Caribbean background. All were, in varying degrees, victims of institutional violence. Although seven of these young adults were obviously autistic, only one had been official diagnosed as such. Perhaps as a result of ignorance, perhaps simply out of convenience, they were labelled as having severe intellectual disabilities. In the absence of proper diagnosis, they were denied access to appropriate treatments and intervention strategies. The response to the severe emotional overload and cognitive frustration that was experienced by those whose autism-related problems were pervasive and intense was inhuman. The characteristic bizarre-like and/or self-injurious autistic behaviour was counteracted or treated by giving these individuals a range of psychiatric drugs.

Michael, one of the young men, was a very intelligent young man suffering from Kanner Syndrome, and should never have been placed in a severe intellectual disability setting, deprived of both intellectual and emotional stimulation. There was very little appreciation in this setting of the hypersensitivities that accompany the condition, and this resulted in either unnecessary restraint or exclusion.

Apart from at meal times there was no real sense of community. Due to the lack of appropriate and basic recreational facilities, many of the young adults simply withdrew to their rooms and lost themselves in compulsive and obsessive behaviours. Stephen, one of the young men I had responsibility for, was over six feet tall and could be violent at times. I was chastised for bringing him in a box of Tic Tac mints whenever I came on duty as it was argued that I was encouraging dependence. Yet that simple gesture was always greeted with such joy. Later Stephen and I would spend many hours making various animal shapes using Tic Tac boxes and plasticine. Stephen was never violent when I worked with him and would always respond very positively when I was sent for when he had been upset.

Brian, a young man with Down Syndrome and autism, was very traumatized, having been abandoned by his family at the tender age of four months. For twenty-five years he had been sent from institution to institution. Brian had an unusual compulsive behaviour disorder in that he would insist on excreting when in the bath. Brian loved having his bath; it was the highlight of his day. Yet some members of staff would insist on his sitting on the toilet for hours on end rather than attempting to modify his compulsive behaviour disorder. Needless to say their efforts were fruitless. I allowed Brian to indulge in his peculiar compulsive behaviour every second day and rewarded his efforts by allowing him to stay in the bath for a longer time on the days he used the toilet. It is difficult to comprehend how anyone could punish such a defenceless and sensitive soul by depriving him of his one and only pleasure, when his compulsive disorder was nothing other than a coping strategy, a cry for attention.

I record the above events from my time spent at this residential home to draw attention to the institutional violence I have witnessed in varying degrees over many years. Such violence is particularly offensive when it is aimed at the most vulnerable of those on the autism spectrum. The members of staff are also affected by this violence. They are asked to cope with situations for which they have not been trained and are largely denied adequate resources. The strain of working under these conditions leads to apathy, which is very often manifested in a combination of ill health, absenteeism and frustration. Great credit must be given to those members of staff who persevere in such adverse situations and selflessly give of themselves in an effort to provide emotional support for the weakest members of our society.

In the sections that follow, consideration is given to a number of elements that I believe are at the heart of the liberation spirituality inherent in the communities at L'Arche. This perspective is also drawn from my experience of working with those at the lower end of the spectrum as a residential care worker.

Honesty

Jon Sobrino (1993) defines the first act of spirit as honesty with the real. 'Intellectually this means grasping the truth of concrete reality.' This act of spirit, this perceptive appreciation, enables us to overcome ignorance and indifference and confront our innate tendency to subordinate truth and to evade reality. We constantly dominate and subvert reality and subject it to our truth, our self-interests, our desires, our violence, our authority. Very often such actions end by imprisoning truth by means of violence and injustice. Concrete realities cease to be living things and become abstractions or mere objects to be manipulated for self-gain. Whereas, '…concrete reality cries no to its own negation to the absence, lack and annihilation of life' (ibid).

Very often those of us who work with, or care for, disabled people are confronted with the unreality of certain educational, social and at times parental expectations. Authority is imposed from above and couched in governmental and occupational requirements that are totally unrealistic. Jean Vanier (1997a) makes the distinction between authority from 'on top' and authority from 'below'.

> Sometimes it is necessary to give orders and clear instructions, to teach, to organise, to show the way with firmness. That is exercising authority from 'on top'. Most of the time in L'Arche, however, we need to call others to life, to help them stand up on their own feet, to help them trust in themselves and their own inner capacity for love. This is

done through our love and compassion; by meeting them where they are, in a heart-to-heart relationship. (p.47)

It is very difficult to meet the needs of those on the autism spectrum when one is constantly subject to the unreality of demands imposed from above, demands imposed by those who are divorced from the reality of the people with autism, demands grounded in socio-economic and/or socio-political expediency. In such an environment both the cries of those on the autism spectrum and those who act on their behalf go unheeded.

Very often the conflict that one experiences with authority is centred on the notion of independence. In a utilitarian culture, if the possibility of progress or success cannot be adequately shown, resources are very often denied, or are totally inadequate in meeting the needs of the person with autism and his or her family. Yet, from the point of view of that person, the criteria for success or progress on offer are alien to the reality of their condition. The failure of those in authority to have a perceptive, sensitive and informed perspective results in misdiagnosis, misplacement and/or the denial of adequate resources. It is not uncommon to find intelligent, non-verbal children and adults with Kanner Syndrome in intellectual disability or psychiatric settings. Sadly, the institutional violence experienced by those on the autism spectrum also extends to their families. Those in positions of authority often dismiss parents, particularly those lacking in self-confidence, financial resources or education. If those in authority were more sensitive to the love, commitment and dedication of parents, carers and professionals, perhaps they would come to a more humane understanding of independence as existentially realized in the struggles of those who work to maintain the dignity and integrity of people on the autistic spectrum. Jean Vanier summarizes well when he writes:

> One of the dangers of society today is overemphasizing people's need for independence and autonomy through competence and strength, and playing down the more basic need of everyone for relationship. We attain human maturity as we live relationships more deeply and become open to others and ready to serve them. (ibid, p.3)

Compassion

The question arises as to how we respond practically to the demands and expectations of those on the autism spectrum and their families. Our response must be one of compassion. It is not enough to observe critically, to be a detached spectator. Life must be suffered. It is compassion above all else that invests us with our human status. Compassion is the primordial act of spirit and the primary and ultimate means of responding to concrete reality. Compassion is a selfless act and requires that we both internalise and participate in the suffering and struggles of others. In *Tears of Silence* Jean Vanier (1997b) writes:

> *compassion*
> *is a meaningful word...*
> *sharing the same person*
> *the same suffering*
> *the same agony*
> *accepting in my heart*
> *the misery in yours, O, my brother*
> *and you, accepting me (p.39)*

If we are to share the sufferings of others with respect, dignity and integrity, 'it is important to approach people in their brokenness and littleness gently, so gently, not forcing yourself upon them, but accepting them as they are, with humility and respect' (Vanier 1996, p.77). Our approach to those with autism must be informed and not one of trial and error. It is for this reason that I have devoted one third of this book to the exploration of some of the central themes and issues that I have encountered, and indeed continue to encounter, in my work with those on the autism spectrum. This is an essential task, a crucial first step. Experience has taught me that compassion is really only possible and affordable to those who have invested time and energy in a comprehensive existential and scientific analysis of the 'Thou' in the 'I – Thou' relational matrix. Compassion, in the context of mutual solidarity and reciprocity, makes possible the transition from being in 'sympathy with' to being in 'empathy with'. It is only in and through our compassion that we can ever hope to be present to those on the autistic spectrum and find the strength to allow those on the spectrum to be present to us, regardless of how broken they might first appear, and how broken we might in fact be.

Presence

Compassion finds its concrete realization in our propensity to be present to the needs of others. In attempting to be present to the real needs of those with autism, there are basically two ways in which we can respond. We can take the 'higher path' or the 'lower path'. To proceed along the 'higher path' is to meet violence with violence. Initial contact with those most adversely affected by autism can be a culture shock. Not only are we faced with people whose reality is very different from our own, but we also have to face the attendant realities of indifference and oppression. Very often we fall into the temptation of acting feverishly on their behalf. We exhaust ourselves in political activity. Such activity can result in exhaustion, ill health and ultimately defeat. Whilst political activity is essential it must be balanced. We lose our balance to the extent that our activity removes us from the everyday reality of those we are attempting to serve. Our inexperience, naiveté, and at times vanity, can result in us responding to authority 'on' and 'in' their terms.

To take the 'lower path' is to acknowledge that the primacy of our task is to listen deeply to the needs of those we serve. In doing so we learn that we are called to 'be' and not to 'do'. 'People need to be reminded that they have not come so much to do things as to learn to be, and that they must not come like a mechanic with tools of knowledge and theory to repair what is broken' (Vanier 1996, p.80). To be doing things constantly, no matter how genuine or urgent it might appear, is first to mirror the utilitarian philosophy of authority, and second to affect the quality of our presence. When working with autistic people, we need energy to attend to and interpret the complexity of their needs. If our sensitivities are constantly being dulled by feverish activity, exhaustion and frustration, we are unlikely to hear their inner cry for love and communion. Furthermore, just as there is no cure for autism, equally there is no solution for the loneliness that accompanies the condition. Loneliness is a reality that must be faced by all human beings. It is therefore crucial that when we are present, we are present without any other agenda other than that of love.

Relatedness

The quality of our presence is in essence determined by the depth of our relationships. Relatedness is the key to spirituality and indeed the central key to the spirituality of liberation. Relatedness to other must be intuitive rather than conceptual, experiential rather than abstract. 'A relation is toward something rather than something. We do not have a relationship but are in relation' (McNamara 1991, p.54). It is not by conceptual knowledge alone, but also by intuition that we come to know a relation. Intuition of self, of other, of the world, of God is primarily experiential.

When working with those on the autism spectrum, we are called to a creative listening. 'A listening to the muted cry that wells up' in the hearts of those we are called to serve (Gutierrez 1996, p.xxxvii). This is a daunting challenge, particularly when faced with people on the spectrum who are non-verbal. Many at the lower end of the spectrum never articulate or express their beliefs systematically. Self-reflection and self-expression are impossible on our terms. Even when working with people who are verbal and/or high-functioning, we are still faced with the challenge of interpreting sensitively the voices of those whose culture and perspective are very different from our own. Yet, if we persevere, we will discover in the presence of the broken:

> ...my friend, my teacher, and my guide: an unusual friend, because he couldn't express affection and love in the way most people do; an unusual teacher, because he couldn't think reflectively or articulate ideas or concepts; an unusual guide, because he couldn't give me any concrete direction or advice. (Nouwen 1997, p.3)

Inherent in the passage quoted above is the notion of transformation. If our relationship with those on the autism spectrum is to be one of genuine mutuality and reciprocity, it must extend beyond the notion of self-transformation. Over the years I have witnessed many people working feverishly on behalf of autistic people, and yet, in spite of the apparent sincerity of their intentions, they remain blind to the hidden presence and beauty of the individual. They fail to perceive that liberation carries with it a contemplative attitude. This attitude is born out of a deep experiential relationship with the inner mystery of that person. The reality and mystery of the individual elicits this response when he or she is taken to be the primary locus of truth. From a Christian perspective, the ultimate truth lies in the incarnational fact of the presence of God in all of reality. Furthermore, 'contemplation is the central human act that puts us perceptively and lovingly in touch with the innermost reality of everything because it is a simple intuition of truth' (McNamara 1991, p.9). The internalisation of the mystery of the Incarnation fosters a contemplative attitude. This attitude is realized to the extent that we creatively select a piece of reality and transfigure and transform it with compassion and love. Contemplation is the means by which we can transcend the relativity of history and the subjectivity of human experience. Ultimately, contemplation provides us with a genuine spiritual context whereby we perceive the mystery of self, other and Wholly Other.

Armed with knowledge and preconceived ideas, many people are inclined to have a vicarious relationship with people who are autistic and are consequently surprised to be initially rejected by them. Yet this hostile reaction is hardly surprising in the light of their sufferings. Jean Vanier (1996) aptly describes their sense of rejection when he writes:

Do not be surprised at rejection by broken people. They have suffered a great deal at the hands of the knowledgeable and the powerful – doctors, psychologists, sociologists, social workers, politicians, the police and others. They have suffered so much from broken promises, from people wanting to learn from experiments or to write a thesis and then, having gained what they wanted – votes, recognition, an impressive book or article – going away and never coming back. Rejected people are sick and tired of 'good' and 'generous' people, of people who claim to be Christians, of people who come to them on their pedestals of pride and power to do them good. No wonder their hearts are closed to new people. (p.78)

When working with people on the autism spectrum, it is essential that we recognize, identify and value the uniqueness and individuality of their humanity over and above their special needs. In *Adam God's Beloved*, Henri Nouwen identifies 'radical vulnerability' as one of the most challenging faces of disability. In recognizing the 'radical vulnerability' of others, we are forced to cope with our own vulnerability. If our relationship to the broken and marginalized does not extend beyond an appreciation of the quality of life we enjoy in comparison to those who are oppressed and marginalized, and extend to a radical awareness of our own vulnerability, we have failed.

One of the unique gifts of both physically and intellectually disabled people is their ability to disarm us of our preconceived notions, our vanity, our pride and ultimately our ego. When working with autistic people, one cannot help but notice their innocence and purity of heart. In spite of their sufferings, they have what Donna Williams describes as a gift to 'simply be', and this in turn challenges us to be likewise. This is one of the most disarming aspects one encounters when working with people on the autism spectrum. They challenge the very fundament of our 'being in the world' to the extent that they open us up to a perceptive appreciation of our own brokenness and vulnerability. Soon we discover, 'we are no different from those we try to serve; we too are broken and wounded like them; …the cry and the anguish of the poor triggers off our own cry and anguish; we touch our point of pain and helplessness' (Vanier, pp.92–3). Inherent in the statements of those who argue they could never cope with either working or living with the broken, is the admission that they cannot cope with their own vulnerability. In a utilitarian culture, the extremity of this admission is, I believe, existentially realized both in the practice of abortion and in genetic engineering.

Unless our relationship with those on the autism spectrum progresses to a radical awareness and acceptance of our own vulnerability, it is doomed to failure. It is not enough to be merely emotionally touched by the life of the autistic person; we must be willing to embrace the reality of being humbled by their presence. Humility is realized to the extent that we allow the autistic person to lead us into a new awareness of self, other and Wholly Other. Humility is essential if our covenant with the sufferer is to be a covenant of mutual equality. Humility not only determines the quality of our presence but it also determines the duration of our presence. Charity may bring us to the door of those weaker than ourselves; humility alone allows us enter. Humility transforms charity to the extent that it transforms a 'compassionate act of detachment' into a 'committed act of love' in the service of others. Humility leads us to a contemplative intuition of the mystery of self, other and

Wholly Other, the mystery of all mysteries. In essence, humility fosters a contemplative attitude, which is at the very heart of liberation spirituality. Devoid of such an attitude, it is unlikely that the 'preferential option for the poor' could ever be realized in a spirit of dignity and integrity.

Communication

At first your picture made no sense,
It had no horizontal lines,
They ran unparalleled
Around vague perimeters,
I was afraid, frustrated.
How could I communicate?

(Adam 1997)

In the lines quoted above, Adam gives voice to the natural sense of fear and anxiety we experience when confronted with the reality of those whose emotional, cognitive and physical impairments disarm us of our standard means of communication. Many people on the autism spectrum are either non-verbal or have limited and/or peculiar verbal skills. A significant number of people with autism also have additional physical disabilities to cope with. Those most severely affected cannot give voice to their feelings, thoughts, needs and aspirations. Yet, in spite of the inability to communicate and socialize in conventional terms, they are capable of forging deep and meaningful relationships. However, the success of our entry into the world of autism, into the possibility of enjoying reciprocal relationships, is commensurate with our ability to learn and adapt to their language.

Communication with the broken is arguably both the most humbling and yet enriching experience of working with those on the autism spectrum. Humbling, in that we are called to value the presence of those considered to be the 'least' in our society and doing so reach a better understanding of our own misplaced self-importance. Non-verbal communication strips us of all pretence. We are robbed of words, which so often reflect the illusions of our hearts. We may deceive and be deceived by words wrapped in various theories and philosophies but we can never escape the silence of our hearts. The word was made flesh. God's self-communication was expressed not in lofty speculative theories but in the body of a man. Likewise, a composer or artist may produce a sublime piece of art, yet that symphony, that picture, cannot say 'I love you'. Communion is achieved in our relationships with others regardless of the risks and pain that this might involve. The depth of our communion in turn determines the quality of our relationships. Henri Nouwen (1997) defines communion as:

> …the to-and-fro of love, where each person gives and each one receives. Communion is a place of mutual trust and respect. It implies humility, openness, vulnerability, a sharing not only of one's gifts and wealth, but also of one's poverty and limits. (p.4)

In spite of the difficulty of adapting and sensitizing ourselves to the subtleties of non-verbal communication, the rewards are vast if we persist. Non-verbal communication bypasses unnecessary social convention and pretence. Stripped of words, we are forced to stand in silence. From the depths of this silence we learn how to attend to the silence of others as the quality of both our listening and seeing increases. This is a creative silence that puts us perceptively and intuitively in

touch with the hearts of others. In silence we hear the primal
cry of those we have come to serve and begin to recognize it as
our own. In the silence of other we perceive the mystery of the
Incarnation and come to know it as our own. In silence we
recoil from the vanity of words and move gracefully towards
contemplation. In silence we refrain from feverish activity,
competition, ambition and from all unnecessary asking and
expectation. In silence we are transformed, as we move from
knowledge to wisdom, from power to vulnerability, from pride
to humility, from security to abandonment and from boredom
to wonder. Transformation comes at a price, the price of
standing naked and exposed to the reality of our illusions. Yet,
as St John of the Cross observes:

> In this nakedness the spirit finds
> its quietude and rest.
> For in coveting nothing,
> nothing raises it up
> and nothing weighs it down,
> because it is in the centre of its humility.
> When it covets something
> In this very desire it is wearied.

(McGowan 1993, p.29)

In a world of mass communications we live in terror of silence,
as is evident in our addiction to television, videos, personal
stereos, computers and mobile phones. Yet none of these can
return us to the very centre of our being. In the silence of
communion with the broken we are transformed to the extent
that we acknowledge their spiritual wealth, and allow them to
lead us to our own. We are challenged to step down from our
pedestals of pride, greed, pretence, ambition and power. We are
invited to acknowledge, not just academically but existentially,

that the 'first will be last and the last will be first'. If, as liberation spirituality contends, the poor and most marginalized have been chosen as the instruments of God's self-revelation, it is precisely because their vulnerability and their pain have humbled them.

Touch

'L'Arche is not built around the word but around the body' (Nouwen 1997, p.34). In Chapter 4, I noted how Adam and Temple Grandin elevated touch to a contemplative level in their work with children and animals respectively. Touch can very often be the primary means of communication when working with those whose autism is pervasive and severe. Situations that call for physical contact such as dressing, feeding, washing and toileting may be the only opportunities we have to demonstrate the depth of our love and commitment. In the passage below, Jean Vanier (1997a) summarizes that which I have experienced time and time again when working in residential care.

> None of these people can speak and most cannot walk or eat by themselves. Each one has felt abandoned. What is important is to reveal to them their value and beauty, to help transform the negative image they have of themselves into a positive one and to communicate to them a desire to live. This communication is essentially through touch, presence and a non-verbal language. One of the most meaningful moments of the day in La Forestiere is bath time, a time of relationship, when by the way we touch and bathe each person we can help each one become aware of his or her own beauty and value. Words are, of course, absolutely vital in some situations as they explain what is being done and

affirm the meaning of certain actions, but the gesture itself is of vital importance...When love is given and received, a trust and peace enters the heart which the face and the whole body radiate. (p.37)

When working with people who have severe cognitive, emotional and physical disabilities, it is crucial we transform dressing, feeding, washing and toileting into moments of relationship. These opportunities for relationship are lost when such tasks are performed without dignity and respect. We perpetuate the sufferers' loneliness and lack of self-worth. We betray them with the denial of our time. We scourge them with the hardness of our touch, our intolerance and our impatience. We crown them with the thorns of their vulnerability. We crucify them with the nails of our indifference. We hide behind 'I could not cope', and fail to recognize their vulnerability, their basic needs, their basic body functions, their cry for relationship and communion as our own. In doing so we diminish ourselves.

Conclusion

In this chapter I have sought to show how relationship and communion are at the very core of the spirituality of autism-related conditions. The spirituality of autism-related problems calls us to an unqualified existential presence. Yet, just as we are called to the presence of those on the autism spectrum, we must allow those on the autism spectrum to be present to us on their own terms. If our relationship with them is to be one of equality, of mutuality, of reciprocity and ultimately of communion, it must be rooted in a spirituality that recognizes the reality of both sufferer and carer. It must be kept in mind, owing to the range of the spectrum, that not all those suffering with autism-related problems require advocacy. Many at the top end of the spectrum are capable of self-reflection and self-expression, albeit at a price. Thus, the spirituality of autism-related conditions is a spirituality for both carer and sufferer (particularly those considered to be at the top end of the spectrum) in that both are challenged to enter into a new and radical relationship.

If we are to embrace the mystery of those on the autism spectrum, we are called to a commitment that is active and restive, contemplative and liberating. We are called to unqualified existential presence, to an adherence of the dynamic principles of experience, of being there for self, other, and Wholly Other without qualification. The spirituality of liberation, as practised in the communities of L'Arche, calls the self to the possibility of a radical and creative transformation of both self and other. In the 'preferential option for the poor' the self is grounded in human experience. Transcendence is realized to the extent that we commit ourselves to the service of others. In our communion with others, and particularly the poor and marginalized, we are called to the mystery of self, other and Wholly Other. More fundamentally we are called to a pedagogy of love.

> To love someone does not mean first of all to do things for that person; it means helping her to discover her own beauty, uniqueness, the light hidden in her heart and the meaning of her life. Through love a new hope is communicated to that person and thus a desire to live and to grow. This communication of love may require words, but love is essentially communicated through non-verbal means: our attitudes, our eyes, our gestures and our smiles. (Vanier 1997a, p.5)

Bibliography

Adam (1997). "Falling to Pictures/Drowning in Words". Unpublished.

Adam (1998). "Diary". Unpublished.

Arendt, Lusia L. (1996). *Living and Working with Autism*. London: National Autistic Society.

Bishop, D.V.M. (1989). 'Autism, Asperger's Syndrome and Semantic Pragmatic Disorder: Where are the boundaries?' *British Journal of Disorders of Communication*, 24, pp.107–121.

Boff, Leonardo (1992). "Spirituality and Politics", in *Liberation Theology; An Introductory Reader*, ed. by Curt Cadorette, Marie Giblin, Marilyn J. Legge and Mary H. Snyder. Maryknoll, New York: Orbis, pp. 236–243.

Bolton, Patrick & Baron-Cohen, Simon (1998). *Autism:The Facts*. London: National Autistic Society.

Cohen, Leonard (1988). *Book of Mercy*. London: Jonathan Cape.

Downey, Michael (1997). *Understanding Christian Spirituality*. New York: Paulist Press.

Eiseland, Nancy L. (1994). *The Disabled God:Toward a Liberatory Theology of Disability*. Nashville: Abingdon Press.

Forrest, Angela, Mills, Richard, Peacock, Geraldine (1996). *Autism – The Invisible Children*. London: National Autistic Society.

Frith, Uta., ed. (1991). *Autism and Asperger Syndrome*. Cambridge: Cambridge University Press.

Gilpin, R. Wayne., ed. (1993). *Laughing and Loving with Autism*. Texas: Future Horizons, Inc.

Grandin, Temple (1986). *Emergence/Labelled Autistic*. New York: Warner Books.

Grandin, Temple (1996). *Thinking in Pictures*. New York: Vintage Books.

Gutierrez, Gustavo (1996). *A Theology of Liberation*. Great Britain: SCM Press Ltd.

Hall, Kenneth (2001). *Asperger Syndrome, the Universe and Everything*. London: Jessica Kingsley Publishers.

Joliffe, Therese, Lansdown, Richard and Robinson, Clive (1992). *Autism: A Personal Account*. London: National Autistic Society.

Jordan, Rita, Powell, Stuart (1990). *The Special Curricular Needs of Autistic Children: Learning and Thinking Skills.* Berkshire: The Association of Heads and Teachers of Adults and Children with Autism.

Main, John (1994). *The Inner Christ.* London: Darton, Longman and Todd.

McGowan, John (1993). *St John of the Cross:Growth through Pain and Sexuality.* Slough, UK: St Pauls.

McNamara, William (1991). *The Human Adventure/The Art of Contemplative Living.* Great Britain: Element Books.

National Autistic Society (1990). *Approaches to Autism.* London: National Autistic Society.

The New Jerusalem Bible (1996). London: Darton, Longman and Todd.

Nouwen, Henri J.M. (1997). *Adam God's Beloved.* London: Darton, Longman and Todd.

Nouwen, Henri J.M. (1998). *Reaching Out.* London: Fount/Harper Collins Publishers.

O'Neill, Jasmine (1998). *Through the Eyes of Aliens: A Book about Autistic People.* London: Jessica Kingsley Publishers.

Schneider, Edgar (1999). *Discovering My Autism: Apologia Pro Vita Sua (with Apologies to Cardinal Newman).* London: Jessica Kingsley Publishers.

Sheldrake, Philip (1995). *Spirituality and History.* London: SPCK.

Sobrino, Jon (1993). "Spirituality and the Following of Jesus", in *Mysterium Liberationis: Fundamental Concepts of Liberation Theology,* ed by Ignacio, Ellacuria and Jon Sobrino. pp. 233–254. New York: SCM Press

Tantam, Digby (1998). *A Mind of One's Own: A Guide to the Special Needs of the More Able Person with Autism or Asperger's Syndrome.* London: National Autistic Society.

Vanier, Jean (1992) From Brokenness to Community. The Wit Lecturers, Harvard University, The Divinity School. New york Mahwah, N.J.: Paulist Press.

Vanier, Jean (1996). *The Broken Body.* London: Darton, Longman and Todd.

Vanier, Jean (1997). *Tears of Silence.* London: Darton, Longman and Todd.

Vanier, Jean (1997). *The Scandal of Service.* Great Britain: Darton, Longman and Todd.

Vanier, Jean (1998). *Community and Growth.* London: Darton, Longman and Todd.

Vanier, Jean (1999). *Becoming Human.* London: Darton, Longman and Todd.

Willey, Liane Holliday (1999). *Pretending to be Normal: Living with Asperger's Symdrome.* London: Jessica Kingsley Publishers.

Willey, Liane Holliday (2001). *Asperger Syndrome in the Family: Redefining Normal.* London: Jessica Kingsley Publishers.

Williams, Donna (1992). *Nobody Nowhere.* Reprinted 1998. London: Jessica Kingsley Publishers.

Williams, Donna (1994). *Somebody Somewhere: Breaking Free from the World of Autism.* Reprinted 1996. London: Jessica Kingsley Publishers.

Williams, Donna (1996). *Autism/An Inside-Out Approach*. London: Jessica Kingsley Publishers.

Williams, Donna (1998). *Autism and Sensing*. London: Jessica Kingsley Publishers.

Williams, Donna (1998). *Like Colour to the Blind: Soul Searching and Soul Finding*. London: Jessica Kingsley Publishers.

Wing, Lorna (1993). *The Definition and Prevalence of Autism*. London: National Autistic Society.

Wing, Lorna (1994). *Asperger Syndrome: A Clinical Approach*. London: National Autistic Society.

Wing, Lorna (1995). *Autistic Spectrum Disorders: An Aid to Diagnosis*. London: National Autistic Society.

Appendix 1

The Triad of Impairments

Social Impairment	Communication Impairment	Imagination Impairment
aloof, indifferent (K)	no communication (K)	handles objects for simple sensations (K)
passive	communicates own needs (K)	handles objects for practical uses (K)
active but odd, bizarre (A)	repetitive, one sided (A)	copies pretend play of others or limited pretend play; repetitive isolated
over formal, stilted (A)	Formal, long-winded, literal (A)	invents own imaginary world – but rigid, stereotyped (A)

Common Patterns of Repetitive Behaviour

complex movements	Kanner
routines involving objects	Kanner
routines in space or in time	Kanner
verbal routines	Asperger
routines related to special skills	Asperger
intellectual interests	Asperger

Abnormalities of:	(i) language (grammar & semantics)	(ii) responses to sensory stimuli	(iii) posture & movement
(iv) sleeping, eating & drinking	(v) mood	(vi) attention	(vii) level of activity

The Autistic Spectrum

Kanner's Criteria	Asperger's Criteria
Profound lack of affective contact.	Socially odd, naïve, inappropriate.
Mute, or language not used to communicate ideas and feelings.	Speech long-winded, repetitive, literal, not conversational.
Fascination with objects, manipulated with dexterity but not for appropriate use.	Poor non-verbal communication.
Resistance to change in repetitive routines.	Circumscribed interests.
Islets of ability, visual-spatial and/or memory.	Poor motor co-ordination and odd gait and posture.
Attractive, intelligent appearance.	Lack of common sense.

Disintegrative Disorder

'Children diagnosed as having disintegrative disorder start to develop normal speech and social behaviour and then regress and lose their speech after age two. Many of them never regain their speech, and they have difficulty learning simple household chores. These individuals are also referred to as having low-functioning autism, and they require supervised living arrangements for their entire lives. Some children with disintegrative disorder improve and become high functioning, but overall, children in this category are likely to remain low-functioning. There is a large group labelled autistic who start to develop normally and then regress and lose speech before age two. These early regressives sometimes have a better prognosis than late regressives. Those who never learn to talk usually have severe neurological impairments that show up on routine tests. They are also more likely to have epilepsy than Kanner or Asperger children'.

(Temple Grandin 1996, pp.47–48)

PDD – Pervasive Developmental Disorder

PDD is the umbrella term used to cover the entire family of autistic spectrum disorders. Within this group, there is a subgroup called PDDNOS (pervasive developmental disorder not otherwise specified) which covers the conditions which do not quite meet the criteria for autism or Asperger syndrome, but are nonetheless in the same family or spectrum.

Other Developmental Disorders	Physical Disabilities	Psychiatric Disorders
mental retardation disintegrative disorder pervasive developmental disorder Down syndrome Fragile X	epilepsy	anxiety
dysphasia – receptive/expressive	hearing impairment	affective disorders – depression, mania, etc.
Dyslexia	visual impairment	obsessive/compulsive disorder
dyspraxia	cerebral palsy	Catatonia
dyscalculia		psychotic disorders
visuo-spatial difficulties		(Schizophrenia?)

Appendix 2

Children of the Bitter Rain

see the children
of the bitter rain
copybook pencil
in a satchel of pain
alone with tears
as buckets of rain
in an ocean of drought

father their eyes
in corners alone
are sticks to our bones
the children of the bitter rain

Clouds of Glass/Vincent's Dilemma

Vincent sits
in clouds of glass
in multiplicity
of orange and yellow
giving his soul
in lost facades
in utterance
of blazing colour

'when you reach
you seldom touch
when you touch
I cannot feel
beyond the fingerprints
on clouds of glass'

'give me a nail
to hang my picture
give me a label
for its title
then take your hammer
to my clouds of glass'

'here, take my ear
that I might feel,
this is my dilemma'

Songs from a Blue Room

you are a child
conceived in a tear
of loneliness

you sit by the water
the swell of emotion to hear
lapping in your soul
you ask
what is it all for

tomorrow you'll be
a teardrop on the sidewalk
playing for lost change

teardrop on a sidewalk
looking for love
passing in the rain

songs from a blue room
this song from a blue room —
for you

Prelude

Read these words as poems
and you will fail,
Read these words as lyrics
and you will fail,
Read these words as prose
and you will fail.

Caste these words
in literary straight-jackets
and you will fail.
Caste these words
in academic straight-jackets
and you will have equally failed.

Read these words as teardrops
passing through the unknown depths
to drown in pools of radical regret.

Read these words as compunction,
the compunction of one lost
to the passing smiles of loved ones and of lovers.

Read these words from one
you have never known,
(or are likely to)
then perhaps you might well draw
some water from the well.

Words and Walls

they gave me words
they gave me walls
as empty as
alarm clock calls

the book of love
the song of songs
they have written
cold iv'ry and ice

my heart is flesh
my flesh is torn
my feet are tired
my bones are sore
you have denied
my child of soul

I knew a woman
mother and wife
bearing the child
of loveless affection

'there must be more to life
than the needle and the sword
the needle threads equality
the sword superiority'

'my heart is flesh
my flesh is torn
my feet are tired
my bones are sore
I find my dreams
in children's eyes'

Touched

as evening fell
he found refuge
in distant hills
far removed
from songs of failing lovers
from the incessant throbbing
of the crowds
he sat with the solitude
of the water and the wood
slowing falling
into silent meditation
he was lost
lost in the emptiness of wanting nothing

when his thoughts returned
he sang a silent psalm
of recollection
'today I have been touched
touched
as by the whispering of the trees
touched
as by the scent of dampened moss
touched
as in the cooling of the stream
touched by a stranger
who came to run her fingers
through my hair
anointing me in oils
with hands empty of intent
empty of conceptual abstraction
another lover
resting in the emptiness of wanting nothing

Saturday Child

Hear that subtle heartbeat
In the silence of your soul
See the mystic waters running
Feel the healing in their flow
Cancel words and reason
So inadequate and vain
And let compassion dance around
The ruins of a Saturday Child

You took the words they gave you
And converted them to stone
You built high walls around you
To protect you from the storm
But when the knave came calling
You were naked and forlorn
The battlements had crumbled 'round
The ruins of a Saturday child

Let the moon kiss your forehead
Let the stars caress your eyes
And if you feel like screaming out
Go right ahead and yell
They say beggars can't be choosers
I say paupers can be kings
So leave the doors wide open 'round
The ruins of a Saturday child

Psalm

I heard the empty wind
call against me.
I cursed the emptiness.
In vain I raised my hands
to push the shadows back.

I looked for you in words.
Words tamed,
Words contained in linear cages.
And I have felt the silent thrust
of rejecting eyes
more cutting
than the words you never spoke.

Now,
I am returning to myself a child,
solitude's child,
a child of solo resignation
threading the thin pencil line
of his existence.
I realise,
it was your silence
I misunderstood.

Davoren

At first your picture made no sense,
It had no horizontal lines,
They ran unparalleled
Around vague perimeters,
I was afraid, frustrated.
How could I communicate?

Today from you a smile,
A pittance of your existence
Would reveal to clumsy hands
The brushstrokes of you collage.
Now I understand,
So let's begin again.

Index